anxiety
toolbox

anxiety toolbox

GLORIA THOMAS

Do you put your life on
hold to avoid the situations
that scare you?

THE COMPLETE FEAR-FREE PLAN

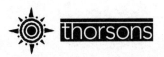

Thorsons
An Imprint of HarperCollins*Publishers*
77–85 Fulham Palace Road,
Hammersmith, London W6 8JB

The website address is:
www.thorsonselement.com

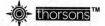

and *Thorsons* are trademarks of
HarperCollins*Publishers* Ltd

First published by Thorsons 2004

3 5 7 9 10 8 6 4

A catalogue record of this book
is available from the British Library

ISBN-13: 978 0 00 717022 7
ISBN-10: 0 00 717022 X

Printed and bound in Great Britain by
Creative Print and Design, Ebbw Vale, Wales

Contents

Acknowledgements

In the writing of this book there are so many people that I would like to thank for their help, either direct or indirect. Firstly, I would like to thank health journalist Sally Brown for an introduction which opened up the opportunity to work with Thorsons, and Dr Roger Callahan, for giving me an incredibly valuable tool as a practitioner in Thought Field Therapy and for writing the foreword to this book. I would also like to thank Jo Cooper who was my teacher in Thought Field Therapy and a great support throughout, and Alexsandra Rehlinger, alexs@artofhealth.org.uk, for her help, especially in anatomy of anxiety. Her incredible knowledge is always an inspiration to study further. Many thanks to Linda Mack for her support and to Nick Johnson, acupuncturist.

Thank you also to my teachers known and unknown who have directly or indirectly helped me get to where I am today. I am very grateful to the originators of Neuro-Linguistic Programming – Richard Bandler, Robert Dilts and John Grinder – for creating a framework of thinking on which to base my work, Ian McDermott at ITS Seminar, Helen Drake at Point Taken and the Atkinson Ball College of Hypnotherapy in Southport. Thank you also to all my clients, because without you I would not have the experience that I have today. The learning is just as much for the practitioner as it is for the client. Thank you to Susanna Abbott for giving me the opportunity to write this book. Thanks also to Jillian Stewart and to Kathy Dyke for the editing. Making the CD was also a very enjoyable experience: thank you to Peter Rinne and Joseph Degnan for making it so.

I thank those close by for their support: Jason Squire, my son Jamie and my mum, Ann Douse. Lastly, I give thanks to God who I believe has given me a role in helping to bring the world back into a place of greater balance through the tools in this book.

Foreword

Anxiety is a very common problem. Anxiety, fears and worry can severely disrupt your life and cause much needless suffering. Research with Heart Rate Variability (HRV) at Harvard – HRV is a placebo-free, objective measure of your state of health – also shows that phobias, worry and anxiety can shorten life expectancy.

Like many people, you may have tried conventional approaches to overcome your fears and phobias and received little or no help. You may feel that you simply do not know what to do to help yourself. This book provides some important answers.

The common motivation to get help and overcome anxiety or phobias is that a cure can radically change your life for the better. Freedom from anxiety makes life much easier, as you can devote your energy to enjoying your family and friends and dealing with everyday challenges, instead of being overcome by crippling fear.

With her book, Gloria Thomas has provided a concise but meaningful guide to various unconventional approaches. She takes a rare, serious, competent and balanced look at some of the lesser-known options that are available and offers an invaluable introduction to them.

Reading *Anxiety Toolbox* is a powerful and appropriate beginning to a new life free from anxiety and fear.

ROGER J. CALLAHAN, PHD

FOUNDER, THOUGHT FIELD THERAPY

LAQUINTA, CALIFORNIA, USA

Introduction

When I was in my twenties and thirties I suffered long periods of anxiety and depression due to a combination of post-natal depression and other life events. Like most people, I sought the advice of my doctor, who prescribed anti-depressants and suggested psychotherapy and counselling. However, much as this was helpful, I wanted to find alternative methods of combating the depressive and anxious states that I was experiencing.

My search for those alternatives uncovered some surprisingly simple countermeasures and some truly astonishing ones. I discovered how beneficial physical fitness is for fighting depression and anxiety, and the surprising extent to which food can affect your mood. I also discovered the benefits of healing and acupuncture, as well as forward-thinking psychologies such as Neuro-Linguistic Programming and hypnotherapy. More recently, I have discovered Thought Field Therapy, an amazingly effective therapy for anxiety.

All of these strategies or complementary therapies – call them what you will – have become part of my life and, as a result, I find myself at 40 feeling youthful, much stronger within myself and with a much more balanced view of life – it's a bit like a giant jigsaw puzzle finally falling into place. Such has been the transformation that I am now incredibly thankful for that period of suffering, for had I not gone through it I would not be equipped to do what I do today. I now have an incredibly strong sense of purpose and, one day, would like to look back on my life knowing that I have contributed to humanity. Given my experience, I feel that the best contribution I can make is by helping people let go of their self-limiting fears so that they can be the best that they can be. That is why I have written this book. It may sound a little cheesy but it's my way of expressing my love for humanity.

There is, I believe, a need for major transformation in this world – a need to get back to more balanced ways of thinking and being. Everybody's anxiety is, of course, unique to them and there is no magic solution for eliminating it completely. However, I believe that we have the most amazing ability to manage our anxiety levels and achieve more resourceful states of mind.

By reading this book, you have hopefully made the decision to begin to let go of fear and anxiety and work towards greater balance in your life. The tools it features are treatments and therapies that are suitable for commonly experienced anxieties, as well as those of a more serious nature. However, I would like to emphasize for those suffering from chronic anxiety or depression that these tools do not take the place of medical advice. They are tools that have worked for me and now I offer them to you. I hope they will help you achieve greater happiness and equilibrium.

How to Use This Book

Whether you suffer anxiety in a very mild form or you have a specific disorder, this book will be an enormous help to you. The intention is to bring your levels of anxiety back under control. You have the potential to achieve states that are more useful and beneficial to your health and wellbeing, and this book can help you achieve this.

I suggest that you begin by reading the book right through to get a feeling of what it is all about and how it can help you. On first reading, do not do any of the assessments or exercises – simply think about what applies to you. Having learned a bit more about anxiety, you can then focus on your own area of anxiety and use the exercises that are appropriate for you. You will need a notebook to do some of the exercises and to record and explore your experiences. Obviously, you will also need a CD player to be able to do the exercises featured on the CD. Although the exercises on it are featured in the book, these were purposely recorded because initially you may find some of the exercises easier to do when the instructions are being read out to you. There are other appropriate exercises and therapies throughout the various chapters of the book, so work through it at your own pace. In chapter 9 you will also find an invaluable summary of exercises and therapies for each anxiety discussed.

What is Anxiety?

Anxiety is a state of mind that we all experience from time to time. I'm sure every one of you can remember having feelings of nervousness and tension in your body at some point in your life – think back, for instance, to your first day at school, your first date or your last vital job interview.

Anxiety is a symptom, a response to a potentially challenging or threatening experience. When the threat is not acute, and we have time to contemplate it, worry and nervousness create anxiety. Anxiety is closely linked to fear, a primary emotion that helps us deal with danger. In an acute emergency we experience fear, and that fear triggers an automatic response in the body that prepares us to stand and fight or head for the hills. However, this natural instinct – which undoubtedly was of great use to our ancient ancestors – is not always useful in today's society, when threats are more often psychological than physical. This means that our bodies prepare us for a physical emergency that rarely occurs.

The only thing we have to fear is fear itself
FRANKLIN D. ROOSEVELT

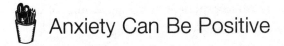 ## Anxiety Can Be Positive

It is important to recognize that some degree of anxiety is unavoidable and indeed can be useful in the short term. It is the body's way of saying 'do this right' or 'pay attention'. In potentially dangerous situations, a lack of anxiety could have disastrous consequences. Imagine walking across the road in the face of oncoming traffic without feeling any anxiety at all. Anxiety ensures that we pay attention to what is important. It is what spurs us on to be more vigilant so that we are prepared for life.

Anxiety can also be a positive experience. Think of a challenge that you have looked forward to in great anticipation – I'll bet you felt some degree of anxiety. You may have called these feelings either butterflies in your tummy or nervous excitement but, either way, they are normal and natural expressions of anxiety – and such feelings can help you to excel.

ANXIETY ENSURES THAT WE PAY ATTENTION TO WHAT IS IMPORTANT

The Anxious Society

Living in today's world can be a bit of an emotional roller coaster and the sort of positive stress that can stimulate and motivate can often be overridden by negative anxiety. The pressures of living in modern society mean our lives are fraught with negative anxiety. Mental distress has now become very common – to the extent that anxiety has been sighted as the most common psychological condition in the UK and US.

There is no doubt that the pace of life these days can be fast and furious. We live in a society that focuses on human 'doing' rather than the human 'being'. We find ourselves on the go all the time and for many of us it's very much the norm to experience ongoing feelings of worry and anxiety as we face the challenges of daily living.

We have so much choice and freedom in so many ways yet we seem unable to exercise that choice in a way that is good for us. We may be wealthier in terms of material possessions – such as nice homes, cars and computers – but we have little time to truly enjoy that wealth because we constantly strive for greater goals and never seem to be totally satisfied with what we have. We have indoctrinated ourselves to live at a pace that falls in with societal expectation. This can bring about anxiety in many different forms. We may be juggling a career with bringing up a family and feel that we must be great at our job, have perfect kids, a good marriage, great social life, great clothes, a good figure … With such expectations, it's hardly surprising we feel anxious! We live by the rules of 'should do', 'have to', 'must do' and seem unable to acknowledge that our anxiety levels are directly affected by how we live our lives.

This sort of pressurized existence, where we are all striving for ongoing individual goals, has also meant that we communicate less with each other. With this comes greater selfishness and intolerance in relationships and increased confusion between the sexes. This adds yet another layer to our anxiety levels.

There are also indirect factors that compound the problem. We are heavily influenced by the media, which constantly portrays the world as a scary place to live – just think of all the headlines about rising crime rates, child abductions, acts of terrorism, war and famine. We are also a society that tends to focus on what does not work, rather than what does work, so it's easy to become hypnotized on a daily basis by the negativity around us. This isn't just bad for our mental health – when anxiety levels rise inordinately it can have a toxic effect on both body and mind.

Worry

Worry is at the very heart of anxiety and is one of its biggest contributors. Anxious feelings often come from worrisome, automatic thoughts combined with the physiological responses that such thoughts cause. Obviously, having the odd worrisome thought is perfectly natural. However, ongoing or intense worry that is repetitive in nature can have a detrimental effect both mentally and physically. When feelings of worry escalate and everything in life is seen as a potential catastrophe, this will start to sabotage an individual's performance in many areas of life.

If you are continuously finding yourself fearful – you are constantly irritable with an ongoing feeling of life being out of control – then you need to begin addressing your anxiety levels. If you don't, constant worrying will increasingly interfere with your life.

WORRY AND ANXIETY CAN STOP YOU ACHIEVING THE LIFE THAT YOU WANT

Individual Attitudes

Given what I have said about the pressures of modern-day living, you could be forgiven for coming to the conclusion that anxiety is a natural response to the society that we live in. However, your levels of anxiety are very much dependant upon you and how you live your life. The way you perceive and interpret events in your life has a profound effect on your state of mind.

Your anxiety levels are determined to a great extent by the beliefs and assumptions that you have about yourself and the world around you.

Those beliefs influence how you respond and deal with threats and challenges and hence how anxious you become.

Some people seem to 'wear' an underlying state of anxiety every day. For others, certain triggers will create anxiety. For others still, anxiety can come about for no reason at all. Your attitude is crucial to how you deal with situations. If you have an optimistic outlook on life, you have empowering beliefs and you deal with situations in a positive way then you are likely to experience less anxiety on the whole. If, in contrast, you have a pessimistic outlook, with limiting beliefs and negative assumptions, then you are more likely to experience anxiety.

Age and Anxiety

Anxiety knows no boundaries and can affect anyone, irrespective of age. Many anxious states are rooted in childhood experiences, particularly some of the more serious ones, but anxiety can manifest at any time or can be related to whatever stage an individual is at in his or her life.

Teenagers, for example, commonly have anxieties about their self-image, exams or early relationships. When we reach our twenties and thirties, anxieties about career aspirations, marriage and parenthood can manifest. Our forties and fifties can also be particularly trying, as this time of transition invariably brings anxieties about getting older and all that this entails. When we reach our sixties and seventies, we worry about the challenges of retirement and our vulnerability in terms of health, security and mortality. In addition, throughout our adult lives, most of us are also subject to financial worries, together with anxieties concerning our children and parents.

Now, whilst all this may have just depressed you, it shouldn't. Instead it should emphasize how important it is to develop a healthy attitude to the unavoidable stresses of life. As I've said before, if you deal with situations in a positive way then you are likely to experience less anxiety.

Specific Anxieties

Individuals experience anxiety in different ways, at different levels and in response to a wide variety of stressors. For example, some people appear to have an anxiety about life in general and view most things, no matter how insignificant, as a potential source of anxiety. For others, the source of anxiety may be more precise – for instance, social situations, their health or a trauma that they have suffered. When we come to very specific sources of fear, the list can be endless – spiders, injections, heights, the dentist ...

The point is that our anxiety, and the extent to which it affects our lives, is very individual, therefore it pays to tackle it in a specific way. (In chapter two, we examine the various types of anxieties in detail.)

Anxiety Disorders

An anxiety becomes a disorder when it is consistent, intense and debilitating, to the extent that it disrupts your life. If you have an anxiety disorder, it is likely that you closely associate an experience or an object with danger and fear, and fixate on it. For many, that possibility of danger is exaggerated out of all proportion to the actual threat. As well as having psychological roots, anxiety disorders can also be caused and exacerbated by physical and energy imbalances in the body (we will look at this in more detail in chapter three). The result is anxiety and behavioural responses related to that anxiety.

When anxiety reaches the stage of becoming a disorder, fear can keep the body in a constant state of emergency, causing abnormal physiological functioning and malaise in both mind and body. So how do you know if you may have an anxiety disorder? The following symptoms are common (though by no means offer a definitive diagnosis):

★ Ongoing sleeping problems or feelings of exhaustion and fatigue
★ Consistent over-worrying that seems to wear you down
★ Ongoing difficulty in concentrating, and becoming increasingly forgetful
★ Feeling continuously tearful or panicky
★ Ongoing feelings of intense anxiety that won't go away, no matter how hard you try

You may also experience 'somatic' symptoms such as headaches, breathlessness, rapid heartbeat, holding of the breath or even physical complaints such as skin disorders or irritable bowel.

We will look at the effects of anxiety in more detail in chapter 3, but for now suffice it to say that the growing prevalence of anxiety is undoubtedly having a knock-on effect on our health in general – it is estimated, for example, that around 70 per cent of people who turn up at their doctor's surgery are suffering from stress and anxiety.

Anxiety can manifest in many forms – phobias, panic attacks, general anxiety, health anxieties, body anxieties, obsession and compulsions, and depression. In the next chapter, we will begin to explore the different types of anxiety that people typically suffer from.

Specific Anxieties

In this chapter we will be exploring the different types of anxieties that people suffer from. The aim is to increase your awareness of any anxiety that may be affecting you. By becoming more aware, you can be more specific about what you are feeling and hence begin to work on managing or eliminating your anxiety forever.

The anxiety disorders featured are the most prevalent in society today. However, I strongly suggest that you do not give yourself the luxury of a label. Although the anxieties we will be examining are labelled 'disorders', suffering from symptoms of one of them does not automatically mean you actually have a disorder. It simply means that you suffer from a certain level of anxiety in that particular area. Remember, an anxiety becomes a disorder when the anxiety is chronic and completely disrupts the sufferer's life. This is very different from having a mild anxiety about a specific area of life.

Before we look at the various types of anxiety, let's examine the methods you will be using to measure your anxiety levels.

Measuring Your Level of Anxiety

I have included two methods of measuring anxiety. The first indicates your level of anxiety and is called the SUD (subjective units of distress) scale. This scale is very well known to the therapeutic community and is used to measure levels of anxiety in the moment, as well as to monitor feedback over time. The method measures levels of distress on a scale of 0 to 10: 0–1 indicates no anxiety, 2–3 indicates slight anxiety, 4–6 indicates moderate anxiety, 7–8 indicates marked anxiety and 9–10 indicates extreme anxiety. The scale is used to indicate the intensity of specific symptoms and overall anxiety levels.

As well as measuring your level of anxiety, you will also be recording how often you experience anxiety. This is done simply by noting if you experience the anxiety not at all, a little, some of the time, a lot of the time or all of the time.

These two straightforward measures provide a clear indication of where there is a problem and the depth of the anxiety.

Rather than discard any particular anxieties out of hand, I suggest that you read about each one. You may have a good idea which type of anxiety you are prone to – and, of course, you may feel no anxiety in many of the areas discussed – but reading about them all initially will help clarify what is appropriate to you and may pinpoint a few other areas that you need to pay attention to. I suggest you invest in a note pad or a journal, and, as you work through the sections in this book that are appropriate to you, write down your findings as you go along.

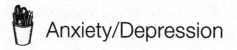 ## Anxiety/Depression

It is quite common for an anxiety disorder to combine with another disorder, and top of the list and most prevalent in the UK and US is the combination of anxiety and depression. A survey by the charity Mind found that 11.2 per cent of women and 7.2 per cent of men in Britain suffer from this condition. Those who suffer from it generally experience a cocktail of emotions, such as hopelessness, sadness, low energy, an inability to concentrate, anxiety, worry, agitation, irritability and restlessness.

Although this book is mainly about anxiety, depression is such a prevalent condition, and one that is so often combined with anxiety, that it cannot be ignored. It is estimated that one in five people will suffer from depression at some point in their lives, and the World Health Organization estimates that by the year 2020 depression will be the biggest health burden next to heart disease.

Naturally, all of us have the occasional day when we feel fed up and pessimistic, but, rather like having mild bouts of anxiety, such moods pass. With depression, however, these moods don't pass and there is a tendency to look at the down side of life most of the time – the cup is always seen as being half empty as opposed to half full. The medical profession defines depression as an illness of both mind and body in which the symptoms are mental and physical. There are obviously different levels of depression and, like anxiety, the seriousness of the condition is determined by how much it affects the sufferer and their ability to cope with life.

The Symptoms of Depression

When someone is suffering from mild to moderate depression, they will feel low physically, mentally and emotionally. They experience feelings of hopelessness and persistent sadness and will often feel they are trapped in a vicious circle that they're unable to escape from. Low energy, tearfulness, a lack of enthusiasm and low motivation are also common symptoms. On the whole, someone who is depressed will view the world negatively and only focus on the bad things in life, and this negative state of mind will be reflected in their body language.

The symptoms of mild to moderate depression are:

★ Inability to sleep
★ Sleeping too much
★ Tears and crying
★ Low mood
★ Loss of interest in things that you usually enjoy
★ Low sex drive
★ Feelings of pressure
★ Concentration and memory problems
★ Feeling muddled
★ Emotional tiredness and fatigue
★ Low energy

If you were to experience the feelings outlined above for more than two weeks then a doctor would almost certainly diagnose mild to moderate depression. With this type of depression, people are often not aware that they are suffering until it is pointed out to them. Do be aware, however, that sometimes such depression can come and go.

If you find it extremely difficult to function properly and your thoughts seem so completely dark that you are almost suicidal then you are suffering from a severe depression. In both cases – and particularly the latter – you should see a doctor.

Self-Assessment
– How often do you experience depression?
– Not at all/a little/some of the time/a lot of the time/all of the time.
– Go through the list of symptoms above and, on a level of one to 10, how much do you experience those symptoms today?

(0–1 = no depression, 2–3 = slight depression, 4–6 = moderate depression, 7–8 = marked depression, 9–10 = extremely depressed)

Different Types of Depression
There are a number of different types of depression, and a number of causes. Reactive depression can occur in response to a stressful or traumatic event, such as bereavement, a stressful job or a relationship problem. An endogenous depression, in contrast, appears to come on for no apparent reason, which can create a great deal of anxiety to the individual, as he or she never quite knows when it will come on again. Bi-polar depression is another name for manic depression, which appears in the form of extreme mood swings between mania and its opposite, severe depression. Seasonal affective disorder, or SAD, is a seasonal depression that is caused by lack of daylight in the winter, especially around January and February. Another common depressive

illness is postnatal depression, which is caused by imbalanced hormones. However, postnatal depression can be psychological as well as clinical, as the mother has to adapt to lifestyle changes as well as the physical changes brought about by motherhood.

As I mentioned before, a large number of people who experience depression also experience symptoms of anxiety. Anxious feelings make you more alert and jittery, whereas if you suffer from depression you are likely to feel that it is an effort to do anything. Anxiety usually precedes depression. However, when anxiety and depression combine, the symptoms overlap.

Symptoms of Anxiety/Depression

★ Feelings of helplessness
★ Feelings of hopelessness
★ Up and down feelings – one moment anxious the next low and depressed
★ Loss of interest in things that you enjoy
★ Low energy and motivation
★ Worry about the future
★ Feeling of being stuck in the present, unable to focus on the future
★ Tiredness
★ Difficulty sleeping
★ Inability to concentrate

Self-Assessment

– How often have you experienced anxiety/depression?
– Not at all/a little/some of the time/a lot of the time/all of the time.
– Go through the above symptoms and on a level of one to 10 how strongly do you experience these symptoms today?

CASE STUDY   for Anxiety/Depression

Viviane was a beautiful 19-year-old who moved to London to make her mark on the modelling industry. She had won all manner of beauty competitions in her home county and it was expected that she would have no problem finding an agent. However, when she got to London, she discovered that life was much harder than she'd imagined it would be. The agency that had been recommended to her turned her down and she found it very hard to get accepted anywhere. After each rejection she found her self-esteem becoming lower and lower. Viviane also had never lived away from home, and she began making do with fast food rather than home-cooked food. The worry about being rejected by agencies was taking its toll on her health. She slept badly and quickly slipped into an anxious depression.

To counter this, I used the anxiety algorithm and the algorithm for depression (see chapter five), both of which worked very well. Viviane and I also worked on her beliefs about herself and she began to learn not to take agency rejections personally and instead see them as simply part and parcel of being a model.

General Anxiety Disorder

General Anxiety Disorder, or GAD, is an anxiety disorder that is characterized by consistent, chronic worry. The American Psychiatric Association has described the condition as excessive anxiety and worry occurring for a minimum of six months. It is estimated that between 2 and 5 per cent of the population of the UK suffer from GAD, while in the US it is estimated there are around four million sufferers. GAD affects both men and women, although statistics show that a considerably higher percentage of women suffer the disorder. Genetics can play a part in GAD, though childhood and life experiences seem to be the bigger contributor.

GAD is a non-specific anxiety, therefore it is not often possible to pinpoint where its roots lie. Excessive worry seems to be present in relation to absolutely everything in life – health, money, job, relationships and even worry about worry itself. With this kind of worry – often referred to as 'meta' worry – life becomes distorted with anxieties about everything. Day-to-day concerns, such as turning up on time for appointments or obsessing over something said or done, are often compounded by daily events on the news and events on a global level, such as the terrorist attack at the world trade centre.

With GAD, worries start internally; the individual starts with negative, limiting and often irrational thoughts about themselves, which develop into an exhausting spiral of negative internal dialogue. Experiences become exaggerated out of all proportion, as the anxiety is always more intense than the situations ever warrant. To make matters worse, not only does the individual with GAD worry about himself or herself, they also worry for their loved ones and anyone else around them.

GAD, at its extreme, escalates to the extent that it causes crippling distress to the sufferer. It can last for weeks or months and seem never ending. To the worrier, it feels as if there are threatening situations and disasters around every corner. If you experience this sort of anxiety excessively then you are likely to suffer other physical symptoms, such as general aches and pains, headaches, light-headedness, nausea, lack of concentration, memory loss and sleeping difficulties, all of which can then create even more anxiety. Like all anxieties, you can suffer from GAD to varying degrees.

Symptoms of GAD

★ Excessive worry about life circumstances
★ Feeling constantly on edge, restless and irritable

★ Inability to disengage with object of anxiety
★ Difficulty concentrating
★ Constant tension in the body
★ Shaking and trembling
★ Being easily fatigued
★ Trouble sleeping
★ Nausea
★ Dizziness
★ Pressure on the chest
★ Sweating, cold clammy hands

Self-Assessment

– How often do you experience general anxiety?

– Not at all/a little/some of the time/a lot of the time/all of the time

– Do you find it difficult to control your anxiety and worry?

– Not at all/a little/some of the time/a lot of the time/all of the time

– On a scale of one to 10, how much do you suffer the symptoms of general anxiety in your life today?

(0–1 = none, 2–3 = slight worry and anxiety, 4–6 = moderate anxiety, 7–8 = marked worry and anxiety, 9–10 = chronic worry and anxiety)

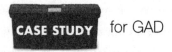 **CASE STUDY** for GAD

Ross, an attractive 24-year-old Australian, was on a travelling trip around the world. Whilst in London, he found himself suffering from severe bouts of anxiety and worry that appeared to be causing on-going migraines and stomach cramps. Ross had a belief that he couldn't cope. These disempowering thoughts were the result of consistently failing exams in childhood and the learning disability dyslexia. When he was in Australia, he was supported by his mother and sister and felt able to manage his life. However, when abroad, he found it

very difficult to communicate his fears and anxieties for fear of ridicule. He seemed to suffer from worry and anxiety about absolutely everything and the slightest thing would cause a negative spiral. He worried about getting a job then he worried about the people around him. He worried that he couldn't get a girlfriend; he worried about his health.

Underlying Ross's worry was a belief that he couldn't cope, so we worked to change this by using some of the beliefs exercises featured in this book. I also used the TFT algorithm for anxiety (see chapter five), and exercises on worry, which allowed him to put his problems into perspective. Ross returned to Australia feeling a lot better.

Social Anxiety

A large number of people have suffered from social anxiety at some point in their lives. Think back over your own experiences and I'm pretty sure you'll be able to recall a period when you were shy and anxious with particular people or groups, or in certain social settings.

To a certain extent, we are born with our personality already mapped out and with an 'emotional' biology that is thought to determine our temperament. Consider babies for a moment – they all have such different personalities. Children born to the same parents also usually have characters that are completely different: one child may have a placid temperament, while another is more robust.

Of course, there is little doubt we are affected by our environment and social anxiety often has its roots in childhood experiences. However, studies examining whether the temperaments of young children changed in social situations over time found that the robust, confident individuals stayed that way in groups of people. The children who were fearful and nervy at an earlier age were more likely to be anxious in social situations, though some did improve.

It is perhaps during adolescence that social phobias and anxieties really begin to manifest and become most apparent. At this stage, children may be breaking some of the bonds with their parents and becoming more aware of themselves as individuals, but they have a strong need to fit in with their peers. As a result, anxieties emerge about being judged or rejected – or indeed doing anything that might conceivably lead to embarrassment or humiliation.

Social anxiety can occur on many different levels. When it is mild, the sufferer usually experiences discomfort and anxiety in particular situations. In cases of extreme anxiety, the individual is consumed by thoughts of their inadequacies and feels quite overwhelmed and panicky. Following a stressful event they will spend hours obsessing about how they could have behaved differently. It is also possible to have phobic reaction in social situations (see page 36).

While the lucky ones grow out of their anxiety, others simply learn to manage it. For some, however, it can stick, causing them to become fixated with self-doubts about social situations. Patterns like this can run the whole of a lifespan and can have an incredibly negative effect on a person's life, making it difficult for them to make friends and get on in social situations. For an unlucky minority, this becomes so fraught with anxiety that they will avoid such situations and hence become reclusive and lonely.

High-tech, Low-value Communication
The computer has patently not helped us to interact with others. Instead of communicating face to face and developing relationships within the family and at work, many of us – kids, teenagers and adults – spend hours in front of the computer, cut off from genuine human

contact. Today, you can, if you choose, virtually lead your life via the Internet – you can do your shopping, click on to chat rooms for conversations and even have a relationship over the net. Dating anxiety is very common, as the insecurities we have about ourselves can negatively affect the way we communicate. Using the Internet can make the initial process less stressful, but of course it throws up many other problems, not least of which are the expectations both parties have built up before they meet.

Social anxiety is often based on perception rather than feedback from others. People with social anxiety become very conscious of the signals that they are giving out and can easily find themselves blushing, tongue-tied or unable to eat, drink or talk; or the opposite – eating or drinking too much to cope with the situation. And, not surprisingly, this can often exacerbate an already difficult situation.

Social Phobia

Social phobia is an extreme type of anxiety (see phobias page 35) in which a phobic reaction can occur at even the thought of being in a social situation. This can escalate into chronic, excessive fear that is deeply distressing to the individual – especially as they are aware at a rational level that the very thing that is making them anxious is harmless. To be diagnosed as a social phobic you must have had the problem for at least six months and the phobia must interfere with your life.

Men and women can suffer equally from social anxiety. In the US, it is estimated there are around 5.3 million sufferers.

Symptoms of Social Anxiety

Do you suffer any of the following symptoms of social anxiety in one or other areas of your life?

★ Worrying about what others think of you

★ Your mind goes blank and you cannot think what to say

★ Thinking about all the things that are likely to go wrong

★ Worrying after the event

★ Feeling inferior to others

★ Self-consciousness and painful awareness of all that you say and do

★ Feelings of panic – heart pounding, sweating and nausea

★ Holding one's breath

★ Speaking quickly, getting words mixed up or mumbling

★ Avoiding catching people's attention

Self-Assessment

– How often do you get anxious and worried in social situations?

– Not at all/a little/some of the time/a lot of the time/all of the time

– Do you avoid the situation that you are anxious about?

– Not at all/a little/some of the time/a lot of the time/all of the time

– Are you afraid of public speaking, giving presentations, and groups of people?

– Not at all/some of the time/a lot of the time/all of the time

– On a scale of one to 10 how strongly do you feel you suffer social anxiety in one or more areas of your life?

(0–1 = none to very slight, 2–3 = slightly, 4–6 = moderately, 7–8 = marked social anxiety, 9–10 = chronic anxiety)

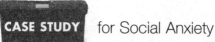 **CASE STUDY** for Social Anxiety

Angus, a 37-year-old marketing executive, works for a well-known mobile network company. Seen as the golden boy of the company, he had amazing sales and marketing skills that brought in a large amount of money. For this he was rewarded with a promotion to the board of directors. One of the respon-

sibilities his new role entailed was holding group meetings and giving presentations to his colleagues. However, Angus had always had an anxiety about his height – he was only 5ft 5 inches – and this seemed to be becoming worse every time he did a presentation. He felt powerless and inadequate, with the result that he mumbled, tripped over his words and behaved in a defensive manner.

In response, I used Thought Field Therapy (see chapter five), a powerful NLP exercise called The Biology of Excellence (see page 206) and self-hypnosis on building confidence in group meetings. And the feedback? According to Angus, the techniques worked a treat.

Panic Disorder

Some people experience anxiety through the feeling of panic. Panic disorders affect 0.7 per cent of the British population and 2.4 million Americans, and are twice as common in women than men.

The attacks of anxiety that are usually experienced with panic disorder can be very scary and can last from 5 minutes to 30. An individual can feel fine one minute and the next find themselves in the grip of extreme fear and anxiety for no apparent reason. An attack is usually preceded by a feeling of something being not quite right. This then quickly escalates into sheer panic, absolute terror and a feeling of being out of control. The catastrophic thoughts that follow the initial sense of foreboding cause a powerful physiological response, which then reinforces the thoughts. It is this feedback loop between thought and sensation that exacerbates the condition, causing anxiety to spiral out of control. At the height of an acute panic attack the sufferer feels completely powerless and really believes that this time the worst is going to happen – i.e. that they are about to die or go crazy. (Thankfully, this never happens.) Some people may only experience one or two panic attacks in a lifetime but others are plagued with panic attacks on a weekly or monthly basis.

Panic attacks can, of course, be mild and therefore will not have a huge impact on a person's life. However, when they are acute and debilitating they can restrict the sufferer's life in many areas. This is due not only to the fear of causing an attack but because of the uncertainty as to when and where the next one is going to occur. Hence sufferers avoid certain situations, places and people that could bring on an attack or where they would feel vulnerable or embarrassed should one happen.

Unfortunately, fear of an attack can often bring on the condition itself. Fear makes us more alert and hypersensitive and we can then begin to look out for any bodily sensations that indicate a panic attack is going to occur or any situations that could bring one on – for example, being in a lift or a crowded room or in an aeroplane, anything that is a reminder of the original attack. Panic attacks can also occur during sleep. The sufferer will waken up gripped with fear, and panic that they are going to have a heart attack.

Like most other anxiety disorders, if you suffer from panic disorder you are also likely to suffer from anxiety in other areas. Depression is closely linked to panic disorder, as is agoraphobia, claustrophobia and social phobia.

What Causes Panic Attacks?

The causes of panic attacks are varied. Personality type can be a contributory factor, as people who are naturally prone to anxiety are more likely to have a panic attack. Sometimes they are born from childhood events, such as separation from parents or one parent. A study showed that rat pups separated from their mothers had greater levels of anxiety than those whose mothers were not removed.

Associating something with other uncomfortable and stressful experiences from the past – for example mental, emotional or physical abuse – is also a common trigger.

Panic attacks do not always have their roots in childhood. Panic attacks can suddenly come on for no apparent reason in adulthood. Life changes and worries about impending life changes are often at the bottom of this, although it has to be said that the possible psychological causes of panic are endless. There are also possible physical causes for panic attack. These include unstable blood sugar levels, hyperventilation and food allergies.

It is important to treat panic attacks, otherwise they could become worse or develop into other disorders. There are a number of different therapies for treating panic attacks so the condition can be managed or overcome – it's just a matter of learning how.

Symptoms of a Panic Attack
Do you suffer from any of the following symptoms at any one time?
★ Churning stomach
★ Heart palpitations
★ Floating feeling
★ Sweating, trembling hands
★ Lump in the throat
★ Nausea
★ Blurred vision
★ Pressure in the chest

Self-Assessment
– On a scale of one to 10, how strongly do you suffer the symptoms of panic attack?

(0–1 = none, 2–3 = very slightly, 4–6 = moderately, 7–8 = marked suffering, 9–10 = severely)

– How often do you experience panic, panic disorder or panic attacks?

– Not at all/a little/some of the time/a lot of the time/all of the time

– Do you worry about having another attack?

– Not at all/a little/some of the time/a lot of the time/all of the time

CASE STUDY for Panic Attacks

Deborah is a 32-year-old mature student with a history of panic and anxiety-related conditions. These had prevented her from completing her education and she had left school with no qualifications and low self-esteem. Having eventually realized her true potential, she decided to study design. However, as Deborah was waiting to sign up for her course, she suddenly felt vulnerable – there were people in front and behind her and she felt so much older than everyone else. Her heart began to palpitate and her stomach began to churn – she felt completely trapped and unable to escape. Her panic levels rose as she became more and more anxious. Although she had always been nervous, this was completely unexpected. Rather than give up her new-found determination to study she decided to seek help.

I treated her panic using the thought scrambler exercise (see page 209). I then used the new behaviour generator exercise (see page 210) to begin to train her brain to work in a new direction. Lastly, I taught her self-hypnosis for confidence and how to visualize her goals for the future.

T Obsessive Compulsive Disorder

If you experience ongoing anxious thoughts that cause you to repeatedly engage in time-consuming rituals, then you may be suffering from Obsessive Compulsive Disorder or OCD. According to the mental health charity Mind, 1.2 per cent of the UK population have an obsessive-compulsive disorder at any one time. Other research suggests that somewhere in the region of 3 per cent of the population have experienced OCD. In the US, it is estimated that 3.3 million suffer from this intrusive disorder. It strikes both men and women equally and often has its roots in childhood. One third of adults with OCD say that their obsessions began when they were children.

A key feature of OCD is the repeated compulsive behaviour that occurs as a result of dwelling on a perceived threat. Confronted with a particular threat, the OCD sufferer will become anxious and unable to disengage from the object of concern. Fear becomes too much to bear and this then leads to compulsive behaviour. This behaviour reduces the severity of the anxiety or the obsession. However, the relief is only minor and so a vicious circle of more anxiety, worry and obsession can occur, resulting in the need to do the compulsive behaviour repeatedly.

Common obsessions are with dirt and feeling contaminated or the fear that some sort of disaster will occur because you have failed to do something – for instance, turn the lights off or lock the doors. Rituals involve things like washing hands, showering, cleaning, checking light switches and turning off taps. With severe cases of OCD, people have been known to wear their skin away or spend hours turning on and off light switches.

Again, like other anxiety disorders, there are degrees of OCD. It can be mild or it can completely disrupt daily life, as hours each day are spent going through the same ritual repeatedly. Even though sufferers realize their behaviour is bizarre and a product of their own mind, they often cannot stop themselves. With milder cases, the symptoms can improve over time without outside intervention but often those with a more serious condition will find it grows worse and completely takes over their life. In an attempt to calm the situation down, some sufferers will resort to using alcohol or drugs – however, this just creates a whole new set of problems. OCD can also lead to other disordered behaviours, such as obsessions with food, which can lead to eating disorders, other anxiety disorders and depression.

The Symptoms of OCD

★ Recurring intrusive thoughts that make you anxious
★ Engaging in any repetitive behaviour – washing hands, cleaning, switching off lights, showering, praying etc.
★ Feeling unable to control both thoughts and behaviour
★ Fear of catastrophe to one's self and others
★ Depressed mood
★ Addictive behaviours
★ Hoarding
★ A need for order and symmetry
★ Repeating words silently
★ Obsessive worries or anxious, disturbing images

Self-Assessment

– How much do you suffer from obsessions or compulsions?
– Not at all/a little/sometimes/a lot/all the time
– Do you have any of the above symptoms or behaviours? On a scale of one to 10, how much do you suffer from these symptoms?
– On a scale of one to 10 how strongly do you suffer from OCD today?

(0–1 = none, 2–3 = slightly, 4–6 = moderately, 7–8 = marked, 9–10 = severely)

CASE STUDY for OCD

Graham was a 30-year-old graphic designer who worked for a number of large websites. He had been diagnosed with OCD in childhood. At an early age, he developed a fear of contamination and used to clean himself and his surroundings obsessively. His obsession and anxiety was so great that he would take his clothes off to eat his meals because he believed that otherwise his food would be contaminated. The last straw came when he and his family went to friends for dinner and he stripped off and sat in his underpants throughout the entire meal.

In a regression, we discovered that Graham's concerns about contamination stemmed from an experience that he had when he was 9 years old. He found a snake and started to play with it. However, an adult screamed at him that the snake was poisonous, took it from him and duly killed it. Graham felt a great sense of responsibility for that snake and developed a belief that in some way he had been poisoned because of it.

Graham responded well to the TFT algorithm for OCD (see chapter five) and we intervened in his OCD strategy and installed a new way of thinking so that he felt satisfied with his cleaning rituals.

Body Dysmorphic Disorder

People's preoccupations are largely dictated by the society that they live in so it's hardly surprising, given western society's preoccupation with appearance, that Body Dysmorphic Disorder (BDD) is becoming more common. This disorder is characterized by a fixation with perceived flaws in physical appearance and the belief that these are in some way repulsive.

Like all anxiety disorders, individuals can suffer in a mild or chronic way, although to receive a diagnosis the sufferer has to experience a great deal of distress and disruption to their daily life. The disorder is thought to affect around one per cent of the population and both men and women can suffer from it. Although it often starts in the teenage years with hypersensitivity about self-image, it can also begin in midlife when we begin to age.

We construct our image of ourselves largely from what we see in the mirror. Of course very few of us like everything we see and may worry to a certain extent about the bits we don't like, but we can usually interpret what we see fairly honestly. However, those with BDD may construct an image of themselves that is hugely distorted. With the more chronic forms of this disorder, the sufferer is preoccupied with their self-image and develops a heightened perception of their 'deformity'. This can be intensely painful, to the point where their life becomes dominated by self-consciousness.

Anxieties about the body typically focus on unhappiness at the shape or size of body parts and can include anything from the feet to the stomach, breasts and hands. However, most anxieties apparently concern the face – noses, eyes, eyebrows, mouth, teeth and lips. Bodily hair is another preoccupation, as are birthmarks and other such imperfections.

It is thought there are a number of causes for this condition. Genetic disposition is one possibility, as this can make an individual more hypersensitive to the disorder – this is likely if another member of the family suffers in a similar way. In more general terms, the roots of a disorder like this lie with the societal expectations that we should all look a certain way. In buying into this and striving to reach those ideals, people often fall short of them and begin to look on themselves with dislike and self-loathing – and this can grow into obsession and preoccupation with the body. The only ones to gain from this are the beauty, health, fitness and dieting industries, which make a fortune out of our anxieties.

Worries and anxieties about self-image can become irrational to the extent that the person develops behaviours such as mirror checking, excessive grooming or shaving, ritual washing, skin picking and wearing wigs, sunglasses and camouflaged clothing. Undergoing plastic surgery is another aspect of this, as are disordered eating behaviours such as food aversion (which can result in anorexia) or binge eating and vomiting (bulimia nervosa), or simply binge eating that results in obesity.

Men Suffer Too

It isn't just women who are anxious and preoccupied with their appearance. A study in the *British Journal of Sports Medicine* claimed that, with the increased acceptance of physical exercise as a desirable activity, men are generally only motivated to exercise to improve their physical appearance rather than their health. A common anxiety for men is being puny and this can develop into muscle dysmorphophobia. This dissatisfaction with the body leads to frequent workouts in the gym in order to achieve a more 'masculine' size and shape. However, although the individual may become highly muscular, they still see themselves as puny. When they feel that they can no longer develop, steroids are taken to boost physique. Other common male concerns are about penis size and receding hairlines.

BDD can take over an individual's life to the extent that they become self-loathing, living in torment that others will notice their 'flaws'. This makes them more susceptible to developing other disorders, such as

OCD, depression and social phobias, and as a result such people can completely isolate themselves in order to avoid anyone seeing their perceived deformity. They believe that true happiness and self-esteem can only be possible if they change their defect. This anxiety disorder is considered delusional, as it is often only the person who is suffering that is aware of the defect – although they are convinced that it is obvious to others too.

The Symptoms of BDD

★ Refusing to accept compliments about yourself and only backing up comments that feed your concerns
★ Anxiety over perceived flaws
★ Preoccupation with body parts
★ Dissatisfaction with body parts
★ Needing constant reassurance about your appearance
★ Believing that something is wrong no matter what anybody says
★ Frequent mirror checking and body grooming
★ Concealment – using wigs, hats etc.
★ A history of visits to a cosmetic surgeon

Self-Assessment

– Do you suffer from BDD?
– Not at all/a little/some of the time/a lot of the time/all of the time
– Do you find yourself obsessing about your self-image?
– Not at all/a little/some of the time/a lot of the time/all of the time
– On a scale of one to 10, how strongly do you currently feel anxiety about your self-image or certain parts of your body?

(0–1 = no anxiety, 2–3 = slight anxiety, 4–6 = moderate anxiety, 7–8 = marked anxiety, 9–10 = severe anxiety)

CASE STUDY for BDD

Roalh is a 29-year-old physics teacher who works in a tough inner city school. He had always been self-conscious about his body size and height but, on taking up his first teaching job, he quickly became concerned that many of his teenage pupils were bigger than him and could physically intimidate him. Unfortunately, his worst fears were realized when he was taunt-ed and bullied by a group of teenage boys and their girlfriends. He was so ashamed that he was unable to stand up to them that he became overly conscious of his size and took up martial arts and bodybuilding. Even though he reached a size that would have been foreboding to the most ferocious youngster he was not satisfied and turned to steroids and other methods of mak-ing himself look stronger.

In order to treat his obsession with his body I carried out the appropriate TFT treatment (see chapter five). We then explored his beliefs and focused on working towards self-acceptance.

Phobias

A phobia is an intense and persistent fear or aversion for a specific object or situation that poses little or no danger. It is estimated that 1.9 per cent of adults in the UK and around 6.3 million Americans experience phobias, with women suffering more than men.

When an individual has a phobic reaction, they are likely to experience an extreme paralysing fear along with symptoms of panic and nausea. People who suffer from phobias know that their reaction to the object in question seems irrational to the rest of the world – and often they see it as such themselves. However, knowing this makes no difference and, in fact, often only increases the emotional distress and embarrassment the sufferer feels.

Phobias are very easy to identify because of the intense irrational response to the normally harmless, perceived threat. Specific phobias can be about spiders, snakes, escalators, lifts, blushing, visiting the dentist, particular kinds of food, insects, birds, injections, exams, animals, flying, water, blood, needles, heights, tunnels ... The list is endless. There are also more complex phobias, such as agoraphobia, which can be made up of a number of fears.

Like all anxiety disorders, phobias differ in their degree of severity. Some people can manage their phobia simply by avoiding the object or situation that they are phobic to. This is straightforward enough if you have a fear of something very specific that isn't part of your everyday life – i.e. a fear of flying or a phobia about needles. However, certain types of phobia can interfere with life on a day-to-day basis. A water phobia could, for example, not just prevent you swimming but also washing; a phobia about germs can prevent you from ever going outside your house; and a social phobia could have an impact on career choices and relationships.

The cause of most phobias can be found in childhood. Often a state of high emotion is linked to an event or an object or situation, so that whenever the individual finds himself or herself in a similar situation they have the same phobic response. Even the thought of the object or a similar situation can bring on a strong phobic response in the body. Phobias can lead to personality disorders, avoidance behaviours and other anxieties such as OCD.

Symptoms of a Phobic Reaction

★ Intense fear

★ Nausea

★ Hot and cold body temperature

★ Trembling legs
★ Avoidance behaviour
★ Aversion to a specific object or situation

Self-Assessment

– Do you experience extreme fear of one specific object or situation, for example, flying, heights, water, animals, insects, injections?
– Not at all/a little/sometimes/a lot of the time/all of the time/
– Do you feel worried or anxious when you even think about these objects/situations?
– Not at all/a little/sometimes/a lot of the time/all of the time
– Do you avoid the object of your fear?
– Not at all/a little/sometimes/a lot of the time/all of the time
– On a scale of one to 10, how strongly do you currently feel about the object or situation that you feel phobic about?

(0–1 = none, 2–3 = slightly, 4–6 = moderately, 7–8 = marked, 9–10 = severely)

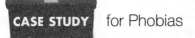 **CASE STUDY** for Phobias

Lesley is a 28-year-old homemaker who has two young children. The children were taught to swim by their father but they were keen for their mother to join in on the fun too. Lesley, however, had a phobia about swimming pools. As a child, she was thrown in at the deep end but, as she couldn't swim, she had to be pulled from the water – much to her shame and humiliation. Lesley never got over her aversion to swimming pools and even the smell of chlorine seemed to paralyse her with fear and nausea. She was terrified that she would not be able to cope if one of the children got into trouble and got upset just at the thought of taking the children to the local pool.

Thankfully, the TFT phobia cure (see chapter five) got rid of Lesley's phobia about swimming pools and she was able to enjoy an outing to the pool with her children.

Health Anxiety (Hypochondria)

Another very common preoccupation of individuals is worrying about their health. Of course we all think about our health at times, but if you experience on-going anxiety about it or obsess about bodily sensations then you may well have hypochondria. Both men and women suffer from it and it can be found in all age groups.

Hypochondriacs are constantly on the alert for oncoming illness and are therefore hypersensitive to bodily sensations and any symptoms of illness. Once they become aware of any symptoms – and they often do find 'symptoms' because they are always engaged in body checking – they blow them out of all proportion.

Those who suffer from severe health anxiety are constantly on the look out for reassurance from the medical profession and are convinced they are physically ill, despite medical reassurance to the contrary. The hypochondriac will pay frequent visits to doctors and often go from one professional to another, never quite convinced by the diagnosis. Often, if the diagnosis is confusing or conflicts with another, they become even more anxious, convinced that there is really something serious wrong with them – a headache becomes a sign of a malignant tumour, a tummy ache could be cancer and so on.

There is a very mixed reaction to this type of anxiety from the medical profession. Some doctors recognize it as a condition in itself, while others are completely intolerant and dread the familiar face of the hypochondriac in their practice.

Health anxiety is more prevalent in western society – which, perhaps, is not surprising. When all your needs are taken care of, you have more time to be introspective and anxious about your health. However, when each day is a battle to achieve a basic standard of living, there is little time to be concerned with irrational worries.

Expressing Vulnerability

Research suggests that anxieties about health are a means of expressing vulnerability. This process, called Somatization, occurs when emotions that we find difficult to express are transformed into a physical expression of the psychological pain. It is now well established that mind and body act as one. Everything you think and everything you feel produces chemical changes in the body. Hence, anxious and worrying thoughts can be expressed through the physical body.

It is thought that this is a very common way for men to express their feelings. Whilst many men refuse to recognize that they are worried or anxious, because they see it as being indicative of weakness, they are much more open to accepting physical illness as a sign that something is not quite right. According to Dr Lipsitt, professor of psychiatry at Harvard Medical School, most of us somatize but people with hypochondria clutch at their physical symptoms to explain why their life is so painful. It isn't the 'illness' that is painful, but the underlying psychological conflict that manifests in physical symptoms. Some anxiety disorders, such as depression and OCD, develop as a result of somatizing.

Illness is also a very useful way of getting support, attention or time out. If, as children, we got away with using a tummy ache or headache to get out of something that we didn't want to do, then we may well use this strategy in adulthood (consciously and unconsciously) to avoid things we don't like or have difficulty confronting. At such times, we can develop aches or pains or suddenly become incapacitated by nausea or a feeling of faintness. People can also sometimes hold on to or develop an imagined illness because it is a good excuse to stop them getting on with their lives.

Of course, the problem with health anxiety is that powerful, worrying beliefs can lead to poor health – they are often a self-fulfilling prophecy. High levels of anxiety and stress create wear and tear in the body. One study, which assessed how the immune system responds to anxiety and stress, found that of the healthy individuals subjected to the cold virus those who were suffering from high anxiety developed a weakening of the immune system and were far more susceptible to the virus than those with lower anxiety levels.

The Symptoms of Hypochondria

★ Spending hours obsessing and worrying about health
★ Never being quite convinced by a doctor's diagnosis
★ Using illness to avoid the challenges of life or to get sympathy from others
★ Thinking that an ache or pain means the worst is going to happen
★ Bodily checking
★ Frequent visits to the doctor
★ A medical cabinet full of pills and potions
★ Frequent hyper-alertness to bodily sensations
★ Fixation and selective attention to bodily events
★ Imagined symptoms of headache, gut pain, dizziness, nausea and fatigue

Self-Assessment

– On a scale of one to 10, how much do you suffer the symptoms of health anxiety?

(0–1 = none, 2–3 = slightly, 4–6 = moderate anxiety, 7–8 = marked, 9–10 = severely)

– How often do you suffer from health anxiety?

– Not at all/a little/some of the time/a lot of the time/all of the time

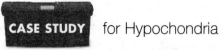 **CASE STUDY** for Hypochondria

Amanda came to see me because she was convinced she had a life-threatening stomach disorder. She had come back from travelling with a tropical disease that affected her stomach, yet despite being cured of this, some symptoms began to return. Her doctor did endless tests, but he could find nothing wrong with her.

Amanda travelled from expert to expert, never feeling that she was getting an answer. When she showed me her medical notes there were repeated statements from her doctors that she was 'catastrophizing' her condition. We spent a few sessions working on her beliefs, as it took some time for her to realize that her illness was a figment of her imagination. I then used TFT for anxiety (see chapter five), and self-hypnosis and visualization to enable her to become more balanced physically, mentally and emotionally.

Post-Traumatic Stress Disorder (PTSD)

Whilst phobias and panic attacks are usually based on distorted or irrational fears, Post-Traumatic Stress Disorder, or PTSD, is caused by exposure to a real-life event that has a traumatic effect on the psyche. When traumatic situations deal your nervous system a real shock, the effects can last for years following the event. PTSD has been described as a normal human response to an abnormal condition. It is estimated that it affects approximately 1 per cent of the UK population and 5.2 million Americans. Women are more likely to develop it than men and it can occur at any age, including during childhood.

The original event that is at the root of the disorder can either be witnessed or experienced. Any reminder of this event triggers flashbacks and severe worry and anxiety. Such experiences can be very traumatic indeed and can be related to everything from witnessing the death of a loved one, to being involved in a car crash or a mugging, or seeing a natural disaster such as an earthquake or an avalanche. It is now accepted that people who suffer from bullying can also have PTSD.

People suffer from PTSD at different levels. If the trauma is mild some people can quickly recover. However, more disturbing recollections and persistent flashbacks and nightmares can take some time to recover from. Any ordinary everyday experiences can remind the individual of the original event, causing them to relive the trauma all over again. It has been suggested that genetics can play a role in PTSD and this could go some way to explaining why it is that some individuals exposed to trauma will suffer only a mild reaction while others develop full-blown PTSD.

Symptoms of PTSD

★ Reliving the traumatic event through flashbacks
★ Ordinary day-to-day experiences remind you of the original event
★ Ongoing nightmares
★ Outbursts of anger and being easily startled
★ Memories of trauma causing significant distress and suffering in day-to-day life

Self-Assessment

– Do you experience any of the above symptoms and, if so, how often do you experience them?

– Not at all/a little/sometimes/a lot of the time/all of the time

– If you have experienced a frightening or traumatic event in your life, on a scale of one to 10, how much anxiety do you suffer every time something reminds you of that event?

0–1 = not at all, 2–3 = very slightly, 4–6 = moderately, 7–8 = markedly, 9–10 = severely

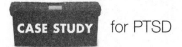 **CASE STUDY** for PTSD

Sunni, a lovely 23-year-old Muslim girl, came to see me in a very distressed state. She had witnessed her mother dying before her very eyes of a heart attack. There was nothing that anybody could do to help her. She felt traumatized by the whole event and was having recurring dreams about what happened. I performed the TFT trauma algorithm (see chapter five) on her. The effect was incredible – one week later, she came to see me and said she felt completely different and much more able to cope. I then worked on helping her to manage her grief and cope with life in general.

The purpose of the self-assessment sections in this chapter is to help you identify where your anxieties lie and at how intense they are today. Irrespective of whether your anxiety is mild or more intense, it can be helped if you carefully follow the instructions in this book. However, this book is not intended to take the place of your doctor – if you are suffering severely, please visit a doctor.

The Anatomy of Anxiety

So where does anxiety come from and why is it so inherent in everyone to varying degrees? It is clear that we all have a biological disposition to feel anxious, nervous or stressed in response to perceived or actual threats. I have already touched on this subject but by examining it in greater detail, this chapter will help you gain a better understanding of why and how you become anxious.

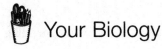 Your Biology

The Central Nervous System

Each of us is a human processing system made up of neural networks that reach every part of our body. These networks are all part of the central nervous system, which consists of the brain and the spinal cord. The brain contains 1,000,000,000,000 individual neurones and can be likened to a computer that controls the workings of the body. The spinal cord, which is made up of nerve tissue and runs from the base of the brain down the spinal column, is like a tunnel running down the backbone. It is not separate from the brain but acts as a highway on which messages travel between the brain and body.

The Limbic System – Your Emotional Generator

The fear response originates in the limbic system, which is towards the back of the brain. This centre, amongst other functions, generates basic emotional responses. These responses are unconscious – in other words they operate out of your awareness. The limbic system is the part of the brain that initially decides whether we should be fearful, angry or loving. It passes this information to the frontal cortex, which is the part of the brain that consciously registers emotion and floods it into our consciousness.

The limbic brain is responsible for the feeling of fear and out of fear comes anxiety. Other primary emotions are love, anger and disgust, sadness, joy, shame, grief and surprise. These emotions are, at their most basic, survival mechanisms that have evolved to help us to run from danger, stand and fight, or move towards more pleasurable states. Although there are a number of primary emotional states, a number of others has developed – for example, frustration, resentment, excitement and so on.

Our emotional states can change from moment to moment depending on what we are thinking at the time. This means we are constantly creating some kind of emotion, whether it is a negative or a positive one. Emotions just seem to happen and it appears impossible to stop them or catch them in the act. Try to control them at a conscious level and you are likely to find it difficult. Emotions are powerful things and at times your emotions can override reason.

The limbic system is made up of a number of structures that work in conjunction to make sense of, and respond to, the incoming information from the world around you: the thalamus organizes the data and information that comes in from the senses; the amygdala, brain's main alarm system, signals and generates emotion; the hippocampus is responsible for storing your memories; the neo cortex is the conscious, thinking part of the mind, whose job it is to make sense of information; and the hypothalamus is the master gland that regulates and controls involuntary functions.

Your Sensory Receiver

Your thalamus is primarily responsible for receiving sensory information and then relaying it to other areas of the limbic system. At any one moment we are bombarded with vast amounts of information. We filter that information through deletion. Can you imagine what would happen if we didn't have a filtering system to erase information? We would suffer sensory overload and very likely go nuts. The information is filtered according to our experience to date. My recent experience of buying of car illustrates how this works. I had never really paid attention to the cars on the road. However, in the car showroom, I was shown a brand new Volkswagen Beetle and instantly fell in love with it. I was amazed that I hadn't seen this car before. I gave myself some time to think about whether or not I should buy it and what happened? I started seeing different coloured beetles everywhere. My new awareness of the Beetle changed the way I was filtering information.

Information That Has Emotional Impact

Information that comes through the thalamus can take two pathways to achieve an emotional response. One pathway leads to the neo cortex, the conscious, thinking part of the mind; the part that explains in detail what is happening – for example, this person is talking to me about a controversial topic. It searches through the stored knowledge for such a thing happening in the past. Stored memories can either come from the hippocampus, which searches through long-term memory banks to make sense of a situation, or the amygdala, which holds emotional information and memories. There is a 'dialogue' about the information and if the brain perceives that a situation calls for an emotional reaction, the amygdale quickly and automatically signals what it perceives to be the appropriate emotional response. In this instance, if you were to have an emotional tie with the topic being discussed then you may react, for example, with apprehension or anger.

However, there is a second route to the amygdala, a much quicker one that can be more useful in times of crisis. With this pathway, the information comes straight from the thalamus to the frontal cortex and amygdala and tells you that you should ACT NOW THINK LATER. This clearly makes greater sense as a survival mechanism, as we don't often have time to have a dialogue with ourselves when confronted with a very real threat, such as an oncoming bus.

The amygdala is the emotional regulator – it decides how much emotional impact each thought carries. Whilst this is excellent in a situation that calls for an instant response, i.e. removal of oneself from path of oncoming bus, there are times when the amygdala can produce completely unnecessary responses that trigger ongoing anxiety. This process, referred to as 'kindling', occurs when repeated stimulus encourage the neurons in the brain to fire excessively, even when the stimulus is not potentially dangerous (see Sensitization, page 61). This response can cause havoc, as stress hormones are constantly pumped into the body, affecting all its major systems – the cardiovascular system, the endocrine system and the elimination system.

We can see that some people are naturally more reactionary and will quickly respond to an experience with fear and anxiety, while others are able to think a little before responding. However, the point is that we can make choices and as long as the perceived threat is less frightening than imagined then, through the use of language and other strategies, you can change your attitude or perception to dissipate a situation. In contrast, if you continue to repeat the response of reacting with fear when it isn't warranted, the result can often be a more permanent state of arousal and higher levels of anxiety.

The Autonomic Nervous System

There is very much a physical reality to our anxiety levels. Anxious thoughts create high states of arousal that have an effect on the natural mechanisms of the body. As you read over the following section think about your own experience and the mixture of physiological responses that occur as a result of your anxiety.

The autonomic nervous system regulates our involuntary bodily functions – i.e. those we are unconscious of. It is divided into two systems that work in opposition to each other – the sympathetic and the parasympathetic nervous systems.

The Sympathetic Nervous System

One of the prime objectives of the sympathetic system is to do whatever is necessary to mobilize the body to handle danger. It is the chief mediator of the body's immediate alarm reaction. Sympathetic nerves originate from cells in the spinal chord and branch out to the rest of the body's organs and tissue sites.

If the amygdala senses trouble, it sends a message to the hypothalamus, a vital part of the sympathetic nervous system. This small but powerful gland is the link between the autonomic nervous system and other endocrine glands (glands that secrete hormones directly into the bloodstream). The hypothalamus is the controller of the involuntary functions of the body, regulating your digestive system, respiratory system, endocrine system and reproductive system. It regulates the hormones involved in governing peristalsis (the natural movement of the intestinal tract), breathing and balance, as well as the heart rate, blood pressure and temperature.

In event of a threat, the hypothalamus relays alarm to the pituitary, another 'master' gland, and the pituitary then tells the other glands what to do – its job is therefore to help produce the hormones that are needed to respond to different situations.

The Three Stages of the Stress Response

The sympathetic changes that take place in response to stimulus are referred to as the stress response. This response was discovered by Canadian endocrinologist Hans Seyle, who demonstrated that the body reacts in the same way to a challenging situation irrespective of whether it is a loud bang, a charging bull, or an extremely pressing deadline.

Selye suggested that there are three phases to the stress response. The first stage is the alarm reaction – your reaction to a given challenge or threat. In response to a stressful event, the pituitary signals the adrenal glands – a small pair of glands that sit at the top of your kidneys – to release the stress hormones adrenaline, noradrenaline and cortisol. Adrenaline and noradrenaline prepare the body to deal with certain conditions and are excreted in times of fear, danger or sexual excitement.

The Effects of Adrenaline and Noradrenaline
★ Your heart begins to beat faster and more strongly
★ Blood flow to the heart is increased
★ Your pulse quickens
★ Blood is diverted to the muscles so that your muscles become tense and ready for action
★ Blood is diverted away from the skin
★ Your breathing becomes shallower and more rapid
★ Glucose is released from the liver into the bloodstream and your blood sugar levels are increased for energy output
★ Digestion slows down to allow the other areas of the body to do their work – i.e. to fight or flee from the situation at hand
★ The pupils may dilate to allow more light into the eyes

If the threat is brief and can be resolved quickly then the parasympathetic system will kick in to reduce stress levels and return the body to normal.

However, if stress is ongoing, you are likely to reach the second stage – resistance. This is when stress becomes detrimental to our health. When stress is ongoing, the result is excessive and prolonged release of cortisol.

Cortisol
Cortisol plays an important part in the stress response and is a key hormone in many other ways – it maintains resistance to such things as

trauma, infections and temperature extremes; it assists in the conversion of carbohydrate to glycogen; it stimulates the release of fatty acids from adipose tissue, which can then be used for energy; it helps to retain the correct water balance in the body; it also counters inflammation and allergies. However, excess cortisol can have detrimental effects on both the mind and body.

The Detrimental Effects of Cortisol

★ Excess cortisol can counteract the body's natural sleep cycles by interfering with the circadian rhythm – the 24-hour schedule that our bodies run to. Normal cortisol levels vary over this period, peaking early in the morning and gradually reducing during the day. Excess cortisol can therefore stimulate the body when it should be asleep.

★ If the level of cortisol is elevated whilst we are asleep, this can also interfere with the body's ability to repair and maintain itself. Elevated cortisol primes the body to use resources; therefore many of the tasks that usually occur during sleep, such as bone and skin regeneration, are postponed. This can lead to poor bone growth and repair, and accelerated ageing.

★ Excess cortisol has a detrimental effect on the immune system, making us more susceptible to viral infections.

★ Cortisol plays a role in depression. It does this by affecting the levels of neurotransmitters in the brain. Neurotransmitters are chemical messengers that are thought to underlie all brain function by carrying information direct to and from the cells. One of the main neurotransmitters is serotonin, which has a positive effect on your mood. If normal levels of serotonin are interrupted by excess stress hormones then you may find yourself feeling blue. Excess cortisol also has a toxic effect on the brain, affecting memory and concentration.

★ One of the functions of cortisol is to break down muscle and convert it into energy when necessary; therefore excess cortisol can lead to muscle loss.

★ Elevated cortisol levels can also lead to excess body fat. When we are stressed the body responds by thinking it is in a crisis situation and stocks up on stores for the future. If you are suffering from ongoing anxiety, you don't eat much and yet you are overweight, excess cortisol may be to blame.

★ Last but by no means least, excess sympathetic arousal of the body, and elevated cortisol, depletes the body's energy reserves. Anxiety uses up more energy than a balanced, relaxed state. If you feel constantly tired, have difficulty getting up in the morning and experience energy slumps throughout the day, this may be the result of excess cortisol.

If stage two of the stress response continues for a prolonged period, with inadequate rest and relaxation to counterbalance it, then the body will eventually reach stage three – exhaustion. At this stage, your adrenal hormones will have been depleted to the point where your tolerance to stress is decreased. In addition, your resistance level will drop and you will experience mental and physical exhaustion.

Read the Signs

You now have an idea of how the stress response can affect you internally – but it also has a marked external effect. Muscles become tense, hence we jut our head forward, hunch our shoulders, frown and may clench or grind our teeth. We acquire different sitting, standing and sleeping postures. We also develop different breathing patterns, often either holding our breath or breathing in a very shallow way.

Pause a moment and pay attention to your physiology. Are you experiencing any tension in your body right now? Are all the muscles and joints relaxed and at ease?

Physical Expressions of Anxiety
Tension in the muscles
Over-breathing

Holding the breath

Shallow breathing

Tension in the chest

Neck aches

Backaches

Heart palpitations

Irritability

Suppression of the immune system

Decreased sex drive

TO CHANGE YOUR STATE YOU NEED TO CHANGE YOUR PHYSIOLOGY

The Parasympathetic System

The parasympathetic system is the other half of the coin that makes up the autonomic nervous system. It is an inbuilt mechanism for counteracting the sympathetic system – it's nature's way of bringing the body back into balance. It does this by, for example, slowing the heart rate down, slowing the flow of air into the lungs and stimulating the activity of the digestive tract and digestive juices. It is also responsible for releasing tense muscles and counteracting the effects of adrenaline. This re-balancing of the body is often referred to as the relaxation response.

In a calm, peaceful body the sympathetic and parasympathetic systems work to retain balance. When one or the other becomes dominant, this is in response to whatever is occurring at the time. When a stressful situation arises, be it perceived or real, the heart will beat wildly, the blood pressure will increase, the digestive system will slow down and so on. However, at some point the parasympathetic must kick in to bring the body back into balance – otherwise you would become ill, exhausted or even die. Unfortunately, because of the stresses of modern-day living, it is the sympathetic system that is mostly dominant, as its purpose is to ensure we survive any immediate threats – and, as we've discovered, we can perceive many things as a threat.

However, if we do not attempt to redress this and pay due attention to the role of the relaxation response – which seems to have been relegated to the role of playing catch-up – then problems are inevitable at some stage. This is because in addition to re-balancing the body, parasympathetic activity is at the heart of many of the body's natural healing systems. Therefore if stress dominates, there is less time for maintenance or repair.

The objective of this book is to bring the body back into balance through promoting activity that will minimize anxiety and promote the relaxation response. Thousands of years ago, medicine men would put people into a trance and tell them that they would be healed when they awoke. In reality, they were promoting the relaxation response and giving powerful suggestions to heal the body and bring it back into balance. It's time modern society recognized the value of bringing this balance back into our lives.

EXERCISE TRIGGERING RELAXATION

This exercise stimulates the parasympathetic system into action to trigger the relaxation response.

Sitting in a comfortable position, begin by focusing on the breath, inhaling through the nose and exhaling through the mouth. Find a spot in front of you that you can look at (you can, if you wish, use a bright piece of sticky paper placed on the wall). Begin to focus on the spot. As you focus on the spot allow your awareness to expand out to the room around you. Whilst continuing to focus on the spot, try and bring your awareness to the back of your head. Be aware of how you feel right now. Experience feelings of calm flowing through your system. Practise this exercise as often as you can.

7   Your Genes

Studies have shown that our genes play a role in the development of anxiety. One in five babies, for instance, are born with a timid temperament. Studies have also explored how genetics affect brain structure in relation to PTSD. Apparently the hippocampus tends to be smaller in people who have suffered PTSD. Further research is being done to establish why this may be: is it because those with a smaller hippocampus respond more sensitively to trauma or is it because the trauma at the root of the PTSD has made the hippocampus smaller?

Further studies have also shown that genes play a role in panic disorder and social anxiety. A recent study at the University of Essex found that anxious people took longer to register information flashed up next to a picture of an angry face than when the faces were neutral or happy. The theory is that anxious people have a much more sensitive fear detection system in the brain. They therefore not only respond to threats more quickly and easily, but also dwell on them for longer than a non-anxious person.

What we are born with is important, but we mustn't overlook the power of our early conditioning to influence our attitude to life. In their first years, babies are constantly learning and responding to the reactions of others. They pick up on their fears and anxieties. If your childhood was miserable and you have anxious, limiting beliefs about yourself you may well have created an arousal system that responds quicker to perceived dangers. If you are in a constant state of high anxiety this can wear down your nervous system and create ongoing tension so that the body is in a constant state of sensitization.

EXERCISE – EXPLORATION

Is there an 'anxious gene' in your family? Does anybody in your family suffer anxious or depressive illness? If so, how do they cope with their condition? Think about your own upbringing – was it positive or negative? What effect has it had on your anxiety levels today?

A Conditioned Response

Having explored how and why the brain produces fear, you can hopefully now understand why emotional states can be so powerful – irrespective of the threat. What dumbfounds many people is the fact that experiences from their distant past can still cause them to consistently respond to sensory stimulus in a certain way. Although you may not be aware of it, over time you train your brain to automatically respond to the sensory stimuli that you pay attention to. It is these automatic responses that trigger different emotional states of mind. This works in the same way as flicking a switch to turn on a light.

With advances in modern technology, science now has the resources to watch the living brain at work. Because of this, much has been learned that can help us manage anxiety in all its forms. It is now widely understood that every experience leaves its mark on the brain. Experiences that create high states of anxiety are produced in the amygdala, and any remotely similar or remembered experiences can trigger a measure of the original reaction. Every time an experience is repeated then the mark is strengthened.

This so-called conditioned response was originally discovered at the turn of the last century by the Russian physiologist Ivan Pavlov (1849–1936). Pavlov discovered that he could trigger salivation in his laboratory dogs by using a stimulus other than food. When he first began his experiments, Pavlov rang a bell and at the same time fed the dogs. He repeated this a number of times. He then rang the bell but did not offer the food. Despite this, the dogs' digestive juices were triggered and they salivated in anticipation of the food. The dogs associated the bell with food and the brain and body responded. The bell had the same effect, even when the dogs were not hungry and even when, time and time again, they were not given anything to eat. And, just like Pavlov's dogs, we respond to the bell or light switch in our mind.

Yet another discovery by Pavlov demonstrated that conditioned responses are more powerful when emotions are involved. High emotions in response to a sensory experience can create a strong emotional trigger that can last a lifetime.

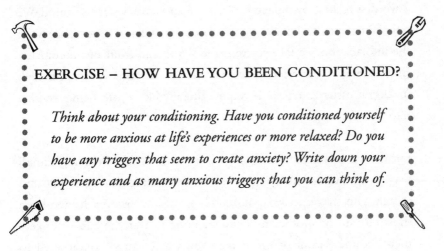

EXERCISE – HOW HAVE YOU BEEN CONDITIONED?

Think about your conditioning. Have you conditioned yourself to be more anxious at life's experiences or more relaxed? Do you have any triggers that seem to create anxiety? Write down your experience and as many anxious triggers that you can think of.

The Pain–Pleasure Connection

Human behaviour is very much influenced by pain or pleasure. Pleasure we are drawn to like a magnet. Pain we avoid. Anything in between the two we tolerate. However, pain manifests itself both physically and emotionally (through anxiety) and we react to uncomfortable feelings by developing 'safety behaviours' that will avert the pain. So someone who is terrified of becoming incoherent in public will focus his or her attention on something else, such as speaking slowly. Someone with social anxiety may avoid making any eye contact whatsoever. For the individual with OCD, continual checking – for instance, for cleanliness or that the oven is off – is very common. Whilst the purpose of this behaviour may be to relieve anxiety, it often preserves the negative thought process that triggered the anxiety in the first place – as a result, each time the situation arises the individual will go through the same response.

People develop safety behaviours to reassure themselves when they are anxious. For many this could be overeating for comfort or smoking in the belief that it is calming. Certain situations or emotions can therefore evoke a reaction that can become habitual through repetition. So a word, a feeling, an image can trigger an anxious state of mind. We train our brains to behave in a ritualized pattern in accordance with the information we take in from the world and from our memories. Every time an experience is repeated the imprint is strengthened, making it easier to repeat. It is quite literally like a path being trodden into your brain.

Further Pavlovian experiments have shown that fear-inducing stimuli need not be consciously registered. Baby monkeys that were put into a cage with snakes showed absolutely no fear. However, having been shown a film of another monkey recoiling in fear, the baby monkeys then became fearful of the snakes. You can become conditioned to anxiety just by watching someone else responding in a certain way.

CASE STUDY

A client told me that as a young girl she had been attacked by a very hungry – and very angry – cat, which flew at her when she unwittingly surprised it. Her reaction was one of complete fear and to this day that same fear is triggered whenever a cat goes near her. However, her daughter picked up on this fear just through watching her mother's response to cats. For many years the daughter couldn't work out why she was so afraid of cats – it was only when, under hypnosis, the link was made with her mother's experience that she was able to let go of her fear.

YOU FIRST CREATE YOUR CONDITIONING THEN YOUR CONDITIONING CREATES YOU

Sensitization

When anxiety is a conditioned response, and the cause of that response is a recurring part of life, it is very easy to become introspective and begin to fear the anxiety itself. Our psychological and emotional state affects our sensitivity to bodily symptoms. Anxiety is a state that does not feel good – it isn't a state to look forward to. For the person who has panic attacks there is always the dread of the next one. For the phobic, the very thought of the response to the object of fear can trigger off avoidance behaviour and anxiety itself.

After repetitive experiences, people commonly put themselves on ongoing alert and hence become ultra-sensitive to their own bodily sensations. When people become sensitized through conditioning they become expert at triggering anxiety at the slightest provocation. In this way, events become distorted and we respond to situations as if we were on an emotional roller coaster. Feelings of fear and anxiety then seem to manifest in situations that wouldn't have previously caused any reaction.

If you experience this ultra-sensitive state, you may find yourself thinking what I call 'sticky thoughts'. These are thoughts that your anxious mind is unable to let go of – they just seem to stick. If you have on-going sticky thoughts you may find those thoughts developing into an obsession or phobia.

Anxiety and Mental Ability

Anxiety also has an effect on your mental abilities. When your mind is rested you are able to think clearly. In contrast, when you are continually anxious and tense, thinking is much more of an effort, you may experience feelings of confusion and find your concentration suffering. Memory can also become impaired. The physical feelings of unease that accompany reduced mental ability are often a good indication that our nervous system has become conditioned to react in a more exaggerated way – and hence that we are suffering from what is termed sensitization. Sensitization is not always a gradual process; it can also come on suddenly as a result of shock, trauma or an illness of some kind. Doctors consider sensitization problematic when it interferes with life. Sensitization relates to the process of kindling mentioned earlier.

The 'Anatomy' of Energy

Since the 17th century, conventional medicine has divided the study and treatment of the mind and body, with each being viewed as separate entities. The result of this is that modern-day medicine excels at surgical procedures and has achieved greater longevity for the individual but the mental and emotional aspects of human health have been widely ignored.

Thankfully, this is changing and it is now widely acknowledged – even in conventional medicine – that mind and body influence each other, indeed that they are inseparable. The recognition of this has come about in part because of the re-emergence of ancient healing systems that, for thousands of years, have treated the human being as one entity. Many of these ancient systems, such as acupuncture, Ayurvedic medicine, reflexology, acupressure and hypnosis (as well as some more recent therapies such as Applied Kinesiology), also embrace the theory that mind and body are not separate from our environment but part of it. The belief is that we operate and interact within a vast sea of energy that never stops transforming itself.

In traditional Chinese medicine, this energy – which they call *chi* – is believed to exist in everything and it is that balanced flow of chi that can keep us healthy and alive. In Ayurvedic medicine, one of the oldest systems of medicine known to mankind, each individual is seen as having a soul energy that links us with each other and with our universe. This concept – that there is really no division between us and the outer world – is far from being 'alternative'. Einstein showed us through physics theory that everything in our material world is made up of energy and, more recently, quantum theory has shown that everything is made up of energy vibrating at different speeds.

How is this connected with anxiety? Well let's see.

Your Energy Body

Every part of you as a human being is energy. Your thoughts are energy, your emotions are energy and your physical body is energy. Every cell in your system is made up out of life-giving energy. You also have an 'energy' body in the same way that you have a physical body. Just because you cannot see it, it does not mean that it does not exist. In fact, as a child you probably were much more aware of energy than you are now. As infants we see, hear and feel the energies that surround people. We all naturally have extra-sensory skills but as we absorb information from the world around us and become older, we lose these abilities through lack of use. The good news is that you can regain those skills by retraining your mind and body to systematically tap in and experience that energy.

JUST BECAUSE YOU CANNOT SEE IT, IT DOES NOT MEAN THAT IT DOES NOT EXIST

The human body is a dynamic energy field. This energy surrounds and penetrates the human body, so each of us energetically interacts with the world around us. The energy field that surrounds the human body is referred to as the aura, which is made up of several layers, called the subtle bodies. There are also seven major energy centres that run up through the centre of the body. These emit electromagnetic energy and correspond with the endocrine system. In eastern philosophy they are called *chakras*, which in Sanskrit means wheel or vortex.

These energy centres have an effect on your physical, mental and emotional well-being. It is said that significant events – both emotional and physical – leave an imprint on these centres. When we become anxious and worried in areas related to a specific energy centre, that centre becomes depleted or can become blocked and congested, which has the effect of directing energy flow elsewhere. This is a fascinating and enlightening subject and I encourage you to explore it further.

The Importance of the Meridians

However, for the purposes of this book, our main focus of attention will be on the energy pathways of the body. These are called *meridians* in Chinese medicine and *Nadis* in the Ayurvedic tradition. These energy highways run throughout the whole body and are connected to and interact with the organs of the body. Meridians also affect every physiological system, including the endocrine system, the nervous system, the digestive system and the immune system.

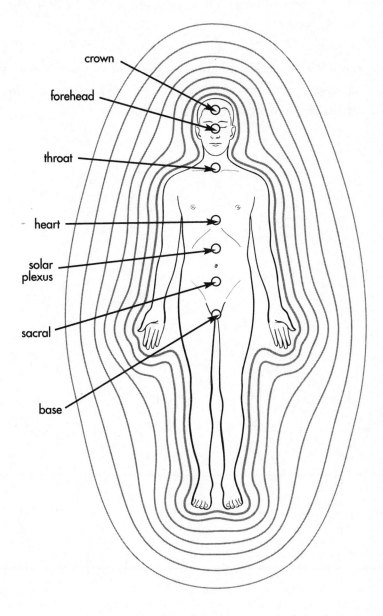

Stress and anxiety can lead to congestion in these pathways and hence have an effect on the major organs of the body. Emotional stress, for example, will affect the flow of energy to the heart, which can create symptoms of palpitations. If energy to the kidneys is affected then fear and lack of motivation can follow. Excessive worry affects the spleen. If you find yourself irritable or angry then the liver is likely to be affected.

Modern-day living makes it difficult to maintain energetic balance in the meridians, as pressure and anxiety can overburden them and affect the functioning of many of the body's systems.

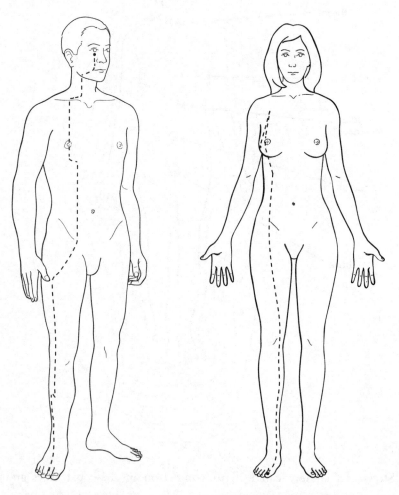

The Stomach Meridian   The Spleen Meridian

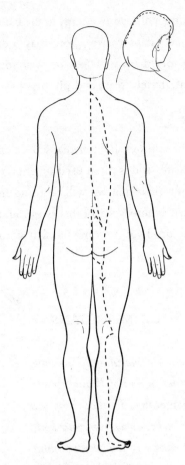

The Bladder Meridian

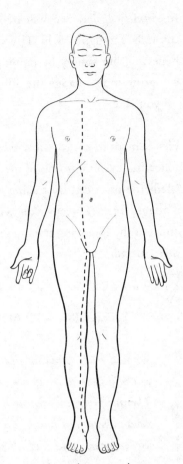

The Kidney Meridian

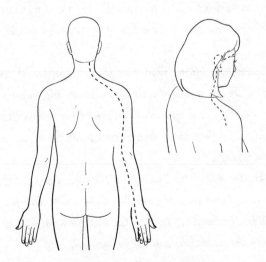

The Triple-Warmer Meridian

In *Anxiety Toolbox* we will be working with your energy meridians through Thought Field Therapy (see chapter five). You may not believe it, but simply by tapping the meridians in a specific way you can profoundly change the affect that anxiety, fears and phobias have on your life.

First it helps to get to know where the appropriate meridians are. The following exercise is one of my favourites and is often used in Energy Medicine practices. By tracing the meridians that we will be using in Thought Field Therapy you will learn where your points begin and end. Do the following tracing exercise until you become familiar with these meridians.

EXERCISE – TRACING YOUR MERIDIANS

We will be focusing on five of the main meridians – the ones you will need to be aware of in order to do the Thought Field Therapy procedures featured in chapter five. To trace them, you need to keep your hands just a few inches away from your body, use an open hand and allow the energy to follow your hand. You can trace the meridian on either side of the body – whatever feels most comfortable for you. Follow the directions given for each meridian and don't move your hand too quickly.

1 *The spleen meridian: Trace this from the inside of your big toe nail, up the inside of your legs, past the hips, up the front of your body. Trace up the side of your ribcage and chest and shoulder and then about four inches down from your armpit on the ribcage.*

2 *The kidney meridian: Trace from the hollow part of the foot. Run your hand over the inside of the ankle and foot then travel up the inside of the leg. Go straight up the front of the body to the point beneath the collarbone.*

3   *The bladder meridian: Trace from the inside of the eyebrow up over your head and neck then go straight down the spine to the sacral joint. Now go over your bottom, down to the knee then over the calf to the ankle and finish on the little toe.*

4   *Triple warmer meridian: Trace from the third, or ring, finger straight up the arm with a bend towards the elbow then go over your shoulder and neck, round your ear and to the temple.*

5   *Stomach meridian: Trace from under your eye down to the jaw, back up the side of the face to the temple then down to the collarbone and down past the stomach, out to the front of the thigh and down to the second toe.*

Now that you have begun to explore the energy in your body, let's look at the part played by your thoughts and emotions.

Your Mental and Emotional Anatomy

Numerous factors affect your physical, mental and emotional wellbeing. In the previous chapter we looked at the physical and energetic influences, so let's now examine how your mental and emotional anatomy play a part in creating anxiety.

The mind functions on many different levels and these influence us in various ways. Your brain has two hemispheres – left and right. The left hemisphere is associated with logic and the ability to analyse and judge. It is time-sensitive and responsible for your intellect. This is our conscious mind. The right hemisphere is the part of your brain that is emotional, artistic, creative and dreamy. It is associated with the subconscious. Both left and right brains are joined together by a fibrous band called the corpus callosum. This band conveys a continuous dialogue between the two hemispheres so that both conscious and subconscious work in an interrelated way. The mind operates at two levels – consciously (with awareness) and subconsciously (out of you awareness).

Making Sense of your World

Human nature is such that we need to make sense of our world. How would we function otherwise? It is the conscious mind that allows us to be aware of our existence. You may have heard the story of the individual who went to see his guru and asked him, 'how do I know that I am?' and the guru answered 'who is asking?' You know that you exist because you are aware of your body and your surroundings.

As I previously pointed out, we have the capacity to take in huge amounts of information at any given time, therefore to avoid sensory overload the information is filtered. I call this part of the brain the executive brain, as one of its main roles is to sort out information,

make choices, analyse, evaluate and judge. Information is then present-
ed to the unconscious part of your mind to be stored with all the other
experiences that you have had in your life. What you see, hear, feel,
taste and smell consciously is represented in your mind through your
thoughts, feelings and experiences. How you interpret this sensory
experience determines your experience and whether that representation is a positive or a negative one.

The conscious mind is also responsible for good old-fashioned
common sense and for making decisions and translating them into
action. It is the goal-setter and behaves rather like the driver of a bus
or the captain of a ship, setting the course and then steering in the
appropriate direction. Your conscious mind allows you to break
down information into small parts. It thinks from the particular to the
general but also from the general to the particular. It compares, evalu-
ates and forms a response to different problems.

The conscious mind is also the seat of our willpower, so it sets the
direction we need to go in to achieve a given task. However, our will
has no power unless the subconscious part of the mind agrees and supports that direction. The conscious mind is responsible for the thinking processes that seem to sit just below the surface of your awareness.
It is also responsible for the voluntary functions of the body, for example opening and closing your eyes, writing, holding a conversation.
Being aware and alert confirms that the conscious mind is active.

EXERCISE – BECOMING AWARE

How conscious of your anxiety levels are you? First explore the external. Take a look in the mirror at your physiology – are you holding any tension in your body right now? Look at your face, your neck, your posture. What would be the signs of anxiety for you – a worried expression, a little frown, clenched fists? Are you holding your breath? Write down your findings.

Now take your awareness inside...

How are you feeling internally? What does anxiety feel like to you? Is it an alert feeling? Is your heart beating faster than normal? Is your mind cluttered, overwhelmed or confused? How often do you feel like this? Is this state one that you experience constantly or is it only apparent in certain contexts? Think about the different anxieties that we explored in chapter two. How aware are you of the intensity of your anxiety? Write down your findings.

Make a commitment to increase your awareness of your anxiety levels. Notice how you respond to certain situations. Be more conscious of how your anxiety is translated into behaviour. If you wish, get a trusted friend to tell you what they think your anxiety triggers may be. You'll be amazed at what you may be unaware of.

ALL CHANGE TAKES PLACE AT A SUBCONSCIOUS LEVEL

In response to the exercise above, recognize that yet another function of the conscious mind is that it enables you to have and make choices.

You can choose if your situation is desirable or not and, believe it or not, you can CHOOSE YOUR THINKING. Your thoughts affect your state and your physiology therefore if you are thinking negatively you can make a choice to think more positively. You can choose more resourceful courses of action. You have more power over your thinking than you imagine. Awareness is the ability to recognize your experience and, if it doesn't suit you, to make the choice to change.

We act out our daily lives in a conscious way. However, the subconscious mind is also at work 24 hours a day, seven days a week to ensure that we function properly. It is responsible not only for the involuntary functions of the body but also for memory storage. Every day you use this part of your mind to recall. The subconscious has also been described as the seat of the emotions – those emotions that pop to the surface in response to a given situation. The subconscious is responsible for your habitual behaviour – the thoughts or actions that you repeat on a regular basis. Your subconscious is the engine to your being, providing the drive and energy to move towards the goals you set yourself. Your amazing creativity comes from the subconscious mind. Awareness of all this activity is a great help in understanding how your subconscious mind is affecting your attitudes and behaviour. Using that awareness, let's look at how messages that travel from deep in the subconscious can affect your state of mind.

EXERCISE – MEMORY STORAGE

Recall a happy event that you experienced 5 years ago. Think about what age you were back then and just allow some memories to pop into your head. See what you were seeing, hear what you were hearing, feel what you were feeling. Now think about a happy event that happened 10 years ago. Now think about 15, 20, 30 years ago.

This exercise illustrates how easy it can be to access your memo-ries and how every experience is stored in your computer-like memory.

Your subconscious mind contains every experience that you have had in the whole of your life. You take in information from the world around you and store it in the subconscious memory banks, ready to be retrieved when needed. Your subconscious draws information from stored experiences. It houses your whole experience of life – the way that you respond to events, your habits, your beliefs. All the nuts and bolts of your thinking are kept in storage. Nothing is ever erased unless the brain is injured.

If a young child, for example, experiences something that causes fear, anxiety and worry, this can lay the foundations for anxious behaviour later on. The event and the feelings associated with it are stored in the subconscious forever. When any similar situations occur, the anxiety from the original experience is triggered.

In their formative years – from when they are born until about the age of seven – children accept everything they are told, irrespective of whether the message is helpful or detrimental. So, for instance, if you come from a family that was fraught with tension then it is likely that anxiety rubbed off on you. However, as adults, we cannot blame our background or parents for our anxiety levels. We possess a free will and can make choices. It is how you interpret an event and what you perceive to be true that will determine your anxiety levels and the choices that you make. Children from the same family all respond differently to situations. What some people find scary or threatening, others don't. Often, if you are unable to deal with a situation emotion-ally, those feelings can become repressed and held out of awareness for your protection. However, as life goes on you may gather similar experiences, often related to the original event. Whenever something similar happens, your subconscious does a scan of those life experiences in memory storage and gives the danger signal to be alert, which creates fear and anxiety.

CASE STUDY

Ruth is a 58-year-old housewife with a life-long history of eating disorders. As soon as she became more than a pound or two over what she perceived to be her ideal weight she would start to starve herself. She would become obsessively anxious about how she looked and would compare herself to others constantly. She spent a fortune on new clothes, cosmetic treatments, diet products and a personal trainer. She just could not accept the way that she looked. She came to me for help because she realized that dieting was causing her to put on weight. Her metabolism was clearly being impaired.

When I did the Timelines exercise (see opposite) with her, a memory came back to her of an event where she and her slimmer sister had been compared and comments were made about her weight. She had felt extreme humiliation. She then took on board the belief that she would always be overweight and set out on a lifetime of dieting to maintain and lose any excess pounds. Having explored her experience, she understood where her fears came from and this understanding allowed her to let go of her fears and change her behaviour.

The following exercise will help you to explore what may be causing your anxiety. I DO NOT ADVISE REGRESSION WORK FOR MAJOR TRAUMAS OR ANXIETIES. I STRONGLY RECOMMEND YOU LEAVE THAT TO THE PROFESSIONALS OR TRY THE TFT TECHNIQUES IN THIS BOOK. ONLY DO THIS

EXERCISE ON AREAS ABOUT WHICH YOU FEEL MILD
ANXIETY AND WHICH FEEL SAFE TO EXPLORE.

EXERCISE – TIMELINES

*Sit back and take a number of deep breaths, inhaling deeply
and exhaling out, until you feel a sense of calm and relaxation.
I'd like to begin by asking you to think about how you organize time in your mind. Think of something that happened a
month ago, six months ago or a year ago. Physically point in the
direction of where the memory seems to come from. Now think
of something that is going to happen in the future – a month
or six months into the future and get a sense of where that is.
Now think about the present and point to where that is. Now
join them all up with your finger so you are creating a line of
time that represents the whole of your life.*

*Close your eyes and bring this timeline to your imagination –
see it in your mind. Now imagine you are floating 100 feet
above the timeline. As you think about your anxieties right
now ask yourself at what other times did you have this anxiety.
Allow yourself to float back along the timeline as events pop up
below you. Make sure that you are floating above the timeline,
looking down on events. Ensure that you are an observer and
that you remain detached emotionally by remaining 100 feet
above – if you experience any feelings float even higher. Now see
if you can float back to the original event but remain completely detached and floating 100 feet up in the air. As you look at
this experience from the position of an observer, what advice
might you give to the younger you that would make a difference
today? What would you rather think instead? What would you
rather feel instead?*

Imagine that you are beaming that better advice and wise counsel to the younger you and watch that younger you receiving it. See the younger you change and transform. Imagine that you are stretching out an imaginary hand so that you have a connection between you and the younger you as you travel back to the present. Experience any differences in how you feel. Travel back along the timeline, taking those words of wisdom and good advice to any similar events that seem to pop up along the way.

Often, simply by exploring your history and gaining an understanding of where your anxieties came from in the first place, you can let go of a lot of them. Many anxieties are the result of negative perceptions of events that occurred in our childhood. We then become stuck with the child-like interpretation we formed at that time. By using the greater understanding and clarity we have as an adult, we can learn to accept a situation for what it really was and hence let go of the child-like fear and anxiety associated with it. This revised perception can allow new behaviours to be installed to create a more positive state of mind.

EXERCISE – AN ENERGY GENERATOR

Think about the times in your life when you had low energy – what were you experiencing? Think about the things you were experiencing in your life to create that low energy state at that time. Take a deep breath and clear your mind. You may need to move around a little to clear any feelings of low energy that remain. Now think about the times in your life when you had optimum energy. As you consider these times, think about what you felt at the time. What were you experiencing to create optimum energy for you? Take a deep breath and clear your mind. Now consider how your state of mind and what you were thinking contributed to your levels of energy back then. How has thinking about these experiences affected your energy levels now?

If the conscious mind is the goal-setter then the subconscious has a very powerful role to play as goal-getter. The conscious mind sets the course and if the subconscious accepts an idea as truth it provides the energy and motivation to work towards the task that it is given. The subconscious mind has been described as a heat-seeking missile – it works to provide the energy to move towards whatever goal it has been given. Its job is to respond to the suggestions that you give it. Once a goal or a suggestion has been set and accepted by the subconscious it can be there forever. For any change to take place you need to convince your subconscious mind. Remember – ALL CHANGE HAS TO TAKE PLACE AT A SUBCONSCIOUS LEVEL.

Most people are completely unaware of this untapped force within and its incredible potential to reach the targets that we set it. People think it is the conscious mind that is in charge but in truth it is the energy from your subconscious desires that is likely to overrule the conscious ones. Therefore, ultimately, it is the subconscious mind that has control and not the conscious mind. If you have been conditioned with beliefs that are optimistic and positive and you aim for success then your subconscious will release its energy to move towards this goal. However, it does this irrespective of the goal. Consequently, if you have been conditioned to be pessimistic and negative, have fearful beliefs and focus on what you don't want, your subconscious will release its energy to work towards that target. Your subconscious mind does not distinguish between positive or negative, it simply does its job. It runs on automatic pilot in response to the thoughts and messages that you give it. Therefore, if you focus on a given situation and worry about it excessively, your subconscious will happily help with manifesting and exaggerating the possibility of danger – unless you can convince it otherwise.

What all this basically means is that your subconscious mind has the potential to generate the energy and motivation for you to move towards the things you want in life. It is the most amazing resource that you could possibly have to steer you towards happier states of mind. This is why it makes so much sense to focus on the things in life that you want, rather than the things that you don't want.

EXERCISE – FOCUS ON THE POSITIVE

Do you focus on the things you want in life or do you spend your life focusing on what you don't want? What effect does this have on your energy levels? If you focus on the negative, make a committed decision to begin to focus on what you want to achieve as you work through each section of this book. Be aware of your energy levels and how they change in response to your new way of thinking. Whenever you feel mentally, emotionally or physically fatigued, you are not using your mind in a resourceful way. Take the time to stop and think about what could be causing you to use your energy in this way – is it fear and anxiety? What can you do to bring your body back into balance?

CASE STUDY

Matthew, a 28-year-old IT consultant, travelled all over the world playing a prolific and high ranking role within his organization. However, the long hours spent flying began to take their toll on him. He was pretty nervous about flying, although not phobic, but he also had ongoing worries about missing his flights. He soon began to get more and more fatigued and came to see me to rebalance his energy levels.

When we began to look at his fears and anxieties about flying, he kept focusing on all the possible disasters that might happen – missing his flight, not being able to sleep whilst on it, something going wrong on board, being stranded at the other end and so on. We set up some simple strategies so that his secretary could organize his travelling time better. We also explored statistics to reassure him that not much was likely to go wrong. We worked through self-hypnosis, rehearsing a positive state of mind and setting up a post-hypnotic suggestion that he would sleep on board. These energy-saving strategies, through simply addressing his worries and focusing on how he would rather be, very soon took effect and he began to feel much better. He found not only did he lose his anxieties about flying, he also began to perform much better in his work because he had more energy.

EXERCISE – CHARGING YOUR BATTERIES

1   *The first step is to breathe slowly and deeply. Now do an anxiety check. Is there any tension in your body now? Be aware of the muscles in your face, your shoulders, the rest of your body – how is your digestion? Take your awareness from*

your feet up to all the possible danger spots in your body. Now take your awareness to your emotional generator – the solar plexus area. Notice any feelings and sensations.

2 *Ask yourself, 'am I ready to let go of any anxieties that are not useful to me right now'. If the answer is yes then focus your attention on the area where you feel most tension and just breathe a positive calm energy into this area. Visualize all the tension leaving your body. When you have a sense that the tension has left, breathe in positive rejuvenating energy to recharge your batteries.*

3 *If there is a part of you that wants to hold on to this anxiety, ask yourself 'what are these feelings of anxiety doing for me?' Wait for an answer and write it down. Now ask the question again. Continue until you get to a deeper level and the underlying need that must be met. Ask yourself how else that need can be met. When you have found the answer, go back to step 2.*

Your Imagination

EXERCISE – USE YOUR IMAGINATION

Stand with your feet hip-width apart and knees slightly bent. Take your right arm straight out in front of you at shoulder level. Focus your eye line on your finger. Rotate your trunk and gently twist as far as you comfortably can. Note the point that your finger reaches. Return to your starting position. Now close your eyes and imagine yourself doing the same thing, but this time going beyond the point that you previously reached. Now allow your body to follow your mind. You will find that you have gone further than you did a moment ago.

The above exercise is a powerful way of demonstrating that we can do so much more than we consciously think we can. Your imagination is so much more powerful than reason, especially when you are experiencing powerful emotions. Yet another function of the subconscious mind is the ability to produce mental images. The mental images that we see come from our memory and imagination. When you make up images you are essentially producing images of what is not present or being experienced. This is the creative part of you, the right brain at work, and it is perhaps the most powerful mental tool that human beings have – the amazing ability to imagine and create our world.

The creative imagination produces works of great art in many different forms. However, imagination is not the preserve of the world's great scientists, artists and musicians. Many people think they have no imagination at all. In fact, that is not true at all – we are all born with a lively imagination. You may simply have suppressed it or learnt to use it negatively. Bear in mind that as children we accept suggestions that we imagine to be true and then act out that imagined truth. Your subconscious mind cannot tell the difference between a real and an imaginary experience.

EXERCISE – TEST YOUR IMAGINATION

Imagine that you are standing behind a sheet of bulletproof glass. Don't just think about it – really imagine yourself in the situation. You know nothing can break that glass. You feel invincible. Now imagine a group of people gathering rocks to throw at the glass. Experience what you feel. Now they begin to throw those rocks. What happens?

I should imagine most of you probably found yourself automatically wanting to duck.

The above exercise illustrates that although logic tells the mind that something is not a danger, this does not prevent feelings of anxiety and tension arising. This occurs when the dominant memory associated with the object or situation – in this case, stones being thrown at glass – is of an inherent threat of some kind. Our need for self-preservation then overrides logic.

FEAR CAN DISCONNECT YOU FROM REALISTIC THINKING

Imagination and Anxiety

So many of our fears and anxieties are a result of how we imagine things to be. We worry about how things are and how they should be and seek to find ways of solving our problems – again by using our imagination. The greatest scientists in the world have always done this. Einstein discovered his theory of relativity in a dream-like state using his imagination, whilst Mozart composed much of his music in his dreams. However, if you use your imagination in a negative way, you will not find a solution. Negative imagination fuels fearful states of mind. Just think for a moment of all the fears and anxieties that you have – I can't do this, I can't see myself doing that, it'll all go horribly wrong ... It's all too easy to blow such thoughts out of proportion and imagine the worst possible scenario.

Our imagination uses both pictures and words and is ticking over all the time. However, the body is perfectly capable of responding to imagined experience as if it were real. Think about how you salivate when you think of your favourite food, how you respond to the sexy thoughts that you have and how you respond to the anxious ones.

It is here, in our imagination and conditioning, that disorders are born. If you imagine all kinds of frightening scenarios when you experience different bodily symptoms, then you create health anxiety. If you imagine there are worries around every corner then GAD becomes a realistic prospect, because problems will just keep popping up. The person with OCD who continually imagines the possible catastrophe if they leave the oven on, will soon become conditioned to check and check again that it is turned off.

All these difficulties are, in fact, self-created. When we focus on negative thought processes we give them the energy to become reality. The very thing we fear can then happen. Often we train our brain to focus on what we don't want and when we do this, what we don't want is often exactly what we get. Once you envision your fears in your mind, your expectation of them can make them happen.

CASE STUDY

Birgit came to see me about the anxiety she felt over giving presentations. She was terrified that she would forget what she had to say and imagined the worst possible scenario happening. When we focused on where this anxiety came from, Birgit recounted an experience she had in a school talent competition at the age of seven. She had not prepared properly for it and when she got up in front of all the parents she was unable to recall what she had to do. She felt humiliated and embarrassed. Since that experience she avoided public speaking as much as she could. When she did have to do it, fear would well up at the remembered experience and her imagination would work overtime to create potential disastrous scenarios.

We worked on creative visualization to enable her to see how she would like to appear to her audience. We also did the Biology of Excellence exercise (see page 206). With an important presentation to give in Australia, Birgit worked on these – she later sent a postcard to say she had given the performance of her life.

EXERCISE – CREATE A NEW SCRIPT

What movies are you running in your mind that are causing and creating anxiety? Think about a situation that makes you anxious.

Now sit back and imagine that you are in a cinema. See a big white movie screen. Now put that situation up on the screen and run the movie of that experience. See what you see, hear what you hear and feel what you feel. As you now look at this experience from the position of an observer, what is there to learn from this experience that will enable you to begin the process of letting go of your anxiety? Using what you have learned, think about how you could rewrite the script – what would you be seeing, hearing and feeling instead?

YOUR IMAGINATION IS ONE OF THE MOST POWERFUL RESOURCES YOU HAVE FOR MAKING CHANGES IN YOUR LIFE

Habits

We have already explored the conditioned responses that create anxiety and how it is that we respond to the 'switches' in our mind. Out of these conditioned thought processes come habitual behaviours, habitual thinking and habitual emotional states of mind. These habits sometimes last for a lifetime.

Habits are a result of the inner dialogue we have with ourselves and the way we have been conditioned to approach life. Although we can develop new habits over our lifetime, they mostly develop in childhood. For example, you have had to learn to walk, talk and brush your teeth – and once you have consciously learnt how to do something then you practise, practise, practise. Imagine how time-consuming it would be if you still had to think how to brush your teeth or climb the stairs. Think about the habitual behaviours you have acquired more recently – driving a car, learning a new skill at work or a sport. There are so many physical skills that we do automatically.

Habits don't stop there, however. Much of your internal thinking becomes habitual over time. You weren't born with the anxieties that you have today – you have learnt them. You weren't born with a phobic reaction, panic attacks or chronic worrying. You have learnt to have these reactions in response to your perception of your experiences. Think of the things that you repeat and say to yourself on a regular basis. These are habitual ways of thinking.

Safety Habits

All habits begin with a single instance of a thought and then an action. Anxiety, for example, can become a habit in response to perceived challenges. As children we are taught to fear things by our parents and teachers. Their actions are, of course, often well meaning and intended simply to keep us safe. So, for instance, teaching a child to be wary of crossing the road is perfectly logical. However, as children we automatically accept our parents' or teachers' suggestions as truth, irrespective of how appropriate they are, and this means we can easily be taught inappropriate responses. A parent who is overly fastidious about dirt and cleanliness, for example, can easily pass their fears about the dangers of dirt or 'contamination' on to their child, who can then develop a disproportionate response to dirt.

Numerous other habitual responses are the result of childhood conditioning. If, for example, you were given a chocolate bar or treat whenever you felt anxious or upset and it made you feel better, it's highly likely that this behaviour will become automatic after time. Hence, as an adult, any time you feel anxious you may head straight for the local sweetshop. Every time the stress response is triggered you do something to appease yourself and move towards more pleasurable states of mind.

We learn to build and reinforce those early behaviours if they give us pleasure or help us to avoid pain. And the more you repeat the behaviour or thought, the more automatic it becomes. Repeated actions become ingrained whether they are positive or negative – remember, the brain cannot tell the difference between the two.

At the root of these behavioural problems are the repeated thought patterns that lie underneath. The more you hold on to negative habitual thought patterns or an ongoing limiting belief, the more expert you become at them. Think about the negative thought patterns that cause you anxiety 'I never reach my deadlines', 'I'm really hopeless at dieting, no wonder I never succeed' – these thoughts become your words and your words become your actions. Your actions become your habits, your habits become your character and your character becomes your destiny. In other words, you wear your habits – they become part of who you are.

Changing the Habits of a Lifetime

Although many people think it is virtually impossible to break life-long habits, this simply isn't the case. They can be changed, if you choose to change them. You have the most amazing ability to move towards more resourceful states of mind.

For some people with anxiety disorders such as OCD, it may be more difficult to stop repetitive actions. However, by exploring your experience to date, you can begin to become aware of the sequence of events that cause your behaviour and hence intervene in the process in the future. It is also useful to put a different frame around your anxiety. Begin to see anxiety as a friend rather than a foe. Experience anxiety as an excited feeling in your body instead of a negative one.

Interrupt your habitual pattern by taking a deep breath and deciding to do something else. Then practise that something else. They say that old habits die hard, but I don't believe this to be so. Sometimes when we try and learn new behaviours and more positive states of mind, old thought processes get in the way. When this happens, the Timelines exercise on page 79 is useful for exploring past experience (always remember to dissociate from the experience when you do this exercise). Once you know when and why you do it, and you know that you want to change a habit, you can choose to unlearn it and create new, positive neural pathways in your brain instead.

You must do the thing you fear and the death of fear is certain
ELEANOR ROOSEVELT

CASE STUDY

Ooonagh, a 38-year-old bank worker, came to see me about her poor time-management. She found it very difficult to get out of bed and be on time for work. She missed buses and trains and was constantly arriving out of breath at work. This was becoming an on-going pattern that her bosses were getting fed up with. She was getting increasingly anxious about her behaviour, as she knew it would only be a matter of time before she received a written warning.

We explored her sleep patterns and discovered that she slept badly. She also drank too much red wine in the evening and ate too much too late – this was her way of relaxing. We explored other ways that she could relax and she came up with a number of new behaviours that she could begin to put into place. We then did the Swishing Away Your Anxiety exercise below, which worked a treat. She read the exercise into a tape and then began to apply it to other behaviours she wanted to change.

The purpose of the following exercise is to begin to train the brain to go in a different direction, by offering it new choices. It is an excellent exercise for changing habitual unwanted states or behaviours.

EXERCISE – SWISHING AWAY YOUR ANXIETY

1   *Think of a negative habit that you want to change.*

2   *Think about how you want to respond differently.*

3   *When you think of the habitual state or behaviour that you want to change, make a picture of it and see yourself in the picture just before it happens i.e. reaching out for the bread bin before diving in and eating its contents. Associate into the picture and experience what you are seeing, hearing and feeling.*

4   *Step out of the picture, take a few breaths and clear your mind.*

5   *Now focus on the state or behaviour that you want to have instead. Make another picture of yourself performing that new state or behaviour as if you had already made the change. Make the image as strong and as compelling as you can.*

6   *Dissociate from the picture and imagine that you are shrinking it until it is a tiny dot in the left-hand corner of your vision.*

7   *Bring back the picture of the behaviour or state you want to change and fully associate into it.*

8   *Have the tiny dot in the corner of your mind.*

9   *When you say the word swish, let the small picture in the left-hand corner get bigger and bigger, while at the same time the present state or behaviour gets smaller and smaller. Do this really quickly. Blank your mind and now do it again five times, each time making the desired state even*

compelling. Ensure you blank your mind between each swish.

10 *Now think about the original state or behaviour. How is it different now? It is likely to be hard to summon that first picture back. If you can summon it easily, swish until you cannot get the original picture back.*

11 *Lastly, test this by imagining a situation in the future. How are you going to respond differently?*

BE OPEN TO CHANGE, WANT TO CHANGE, MAKE A COMMITTED DECISION TO DO IT

CASE STUDY

Ruth, 58, was advised by her doctor to see me. She had spent a number of months at a psychiatric clinic because of a combination of chronic general anxiety and panic attacks. Ruth was completely over-emotional and the slightest thing set her off on an emotional roller coaster of fear, anxiety and negativity. The first time I saw her she appeared to be an emotional wreck – she was shaking and panicky and full of all the catastrophes that were going to befall her in the future. Every sentence was a drama, every word a negative one. However, her anxieties were self-created by her beliefs and assumptions and the negative language she was using.

I used the TFT algorithm for trauma (see chapter five), as she had had a number of real or imagined traumatic experiences. I also helped her to realize that the anxieties that she was experiencing were down to the choices that she was making about her life. The TFT algorithm had the most beneficial effect on her and when she left she was no longer shaking and the trembling in her voice had gone. We also set up some more useful choices for her to work towards in the future.

Your Emotions

The human body acts like a barometer. It gives you feedback via emotions and sensations in response to what you are thinking. The intention is to tell you how to respond to a given situation. Often, if our thinking is emotionally painful, we try and bottle those thoughts and emotions up in order to avoid them. However, emotions that have been suppressed always seem to pop to the surface in some way or other through feelings and bodily sensations.

Every thought you think, every belief you hold becomes a biochemical reality in your body. Any persistent symptom is your own inner wisdom trying to bring your attention to an area that needs compassion.

CHRISTINE NORTHRUP

EXERCISE – WORD POWER

Do this exercise with a friend. Write down a list of emotional states – i.e. sad, happy, fearful, angry. Give your friend the list and ask them to read at random from it. Close your eyes and, as each word is slowly read out to you, notice what feelings come up in response.

Notice that words can have a powerful effect on your emotional state. Make an agreement with yourself to be aware of the language that you are using and of how the language of others can have a profound effect on your emotional state and theirs.

By now you should be aware that many of your anxieties and fears have occurred as a result of the combination of strong emotion and experience. If as a child you were intensely frightened of something and you have established an anchor – something that triggers that original state – then as an adult, no matter how much you rationalize that you no longer need to feel that emotion, when something triggers it, it still seems to override any rational response. Emotions are powerful things; they can override your reason and disconnect you from realistic thinking. The sort of irrational thinking that stems from childlike emotions can play havoc with your life, stopping you from achieving your goals and dreams.

There is little doubt that your past can have a profound effect on your present experience – but only if you allow it to. Although poor programming may have gotten the better of you, allowing your emotions to rule you, you do not have to suffer that programming in the future. You have the ability to handle your emotional state. You can begin by getting to know how your mind works and, through doing the self-help exercises, how you can control it.

AS YOU THINK SO SHALL YOU BECOME

The Nuts and Bolts of your Thinking

We are all thinking machines that never shut down. But have you ever asked yourself what thoughts are and where they come from? Einstein demonstrated that everything is energy ($E = MC^2$). Thoughts have been described as electrical impulses that direct and control us. They emit a subtle type of energy. Every thought you think is energy and they travel through your system activating a physiological response in the body. It's almost like your body is listening in to your thinking and responding accordingly.

The average person has about 50–60,000 thoughts a day. These change from moment to moment and affect your state of mind as well as your physiology. Your thoughts have a structure to them. Their job is to communicate with us – to analyse, organize and structure our lives. Your thoughts are energy and when you focus your attention on something you are directing that energy to a given target. In other words, you are driving that energy to meet your intentions.

It is now acknowledged that we can affect each other with our thoughts, even from a distance. At a university in the US, a study was carried out into the effects of 'distance' healing on individuals suffering from acute coronary conditions. It found that those who were the subject of prayers for healing recovered more quickly than coronary patients who were not prayed for. This is nothing to do with religion. Prayer is essentially a meditative state in which your attention is very focused. Thought combined with intention is a powerful thing.

THOUGHTS CAN SHAPE OUR WORLD EITHER INDIVIDUALLY OR COLLECTIVELY

Self-Talk

They say that talking to yourself is a sign of madness, yet we all chat to ourselves all the time. This mental chatter, or self-talk, takes place just out of our awareness and seems automatic in nature. It is made up of our likes and dislikes, our beliefs and assumptions, and the beliefs and expectations of others.

It therefore goes without saying that the more positive your self-talk is, the more positive and optimistic you are likely to be. Unfortunately, most of the self-talk we engage in is harsh, critical, self-depreciating and irrational.

Think about the things you say to yourself. Here are a few of the things I have caught myself saying recently: 'you stupid idiot you've got it all wrong', 'I can't do that', 'dumbo', 'I'm not good enough', 'everybody is looking at me'. The next time you find yourself feeling anxious and you're unaware of the cause, try rewinding to what you were thinking just before you became anxious. When you talk to yourself you are in fact directing the mind to establish a reality based on that internal dialogue. Think of the different anxieties you have – for instance, 'I'm not good enough to talk in public', 'I know that I'm going to fail miserably at my exams', 'I can't bear to even look at spiders' and so on. All of the negative things that you say to yourself simply reinforce negative states of mind.

This vicious circle of negativity can undoubtedly limit what you do in life, as it creates fear and anxiety. And that fear and anxiety will make you more likely to stick to things that are familiar and 'safe'. Any ex-periences outside of this safety zone are likely to create anxiety.

Self-talk also has consequences at a cellular level. If your internal dia- logue is full of language that creates fear then this has a very real effect on your health. Think of the things you say about your health – 'I feel terrible', 'I know there's something wrong with me' and so on. It's hardly surprising that doctors and medical researchers estimate that around 75 per cent of patients' ills are mind-related.

However, you can learn to intervene in all this negative self-talk by stopping the internal dialogue in its tracks. You can then replace the old dialogue with more useful dialogue instead (see affirmations and scripts pages 172–7).

EXERCISE – DIFFUSE THE NEGATIVE VOICE

Listen to your inner saboteur getting ready to tamper with your efforts to achieve your dreams. Make a point of consciously stopping whatever you are doing. Listen to the voice and its characteristics – whose voice is it? Does it sound familiar to you? (It could sound like a parent.) Alter its tone, pitch and rhythm. Change the content so it is positive. Make the voice funny so that you break into laughter whenever you hear it. Now choose a fun symbol to represent this new voice. The next time your inner dialogue becomes negative, think of the symbol and the reaction that wells up will be a humorous one.

Some of you may think that self-talk happens so fast it is impossible to intervene. The truth is that you can interrupt it if you choose to. First you need to become more aware of your self-talk. The more you get used to listening to it, the easier it becomes to intervene. Once you begin to hear and recognize all the negative dialogue you can stop it in its tracks and change the language that you use to be much more positive. If internal dialogue is causing your anxiety levels to soar, bear in mind that you did not come into the world thinking negatively. You have learned to think negatively in the same way that you have learnt other behaviours. You can choose to unlearn this habitual self-talk and develop new language patterns that will empower you. Once you have changed fear-inducing words to empowering ones, you then repeat those words over and over again until they become true.

There is nothing either good or bad but thinking makes it so
HAMLET

EXERCISE – GET A BETTER PERSPECTIVE

The next time you begin to feel anxious thoughts, explore what is happening. Be aware of the impact that these fearful thoughts are having on your body. What are these fearful thoughts and what is really so terrible about what is happening? What is the worst thing that could actually happen? Ask yourself if it is really likely to happen. Deep inside of you is a place where you can see your thoughts for what they really are. Do you still want to think about those thoughts in the same way that you are currently thinking? What would you rather think instead? Make the decision to take greater control over your thinking processes. Begin with the affirmation I AM IN CHARGE OF MY THINKING and begin to focus on what you would rather think instead.

Remember, you have a choice and if your thinking is not serving you well you need to change it. Next time you have a dysfunctional thought, stop it in its tracks with a word or a smile or clap or by punching your fist in the air... Now choose what you would rather think instead.

The thoughts that you think today can become the building blocks of what you think tomorrow. Those thoughts are creating your attitude, your state of mind – your thoughts become you.

With our thoughts we make our world

BUDDHA

Power Tool 1 –
Thought Field Therapy

One of the greatest motivations for me to write a self-help anxiety book was the discovery of an effective therapy that can help individuals eliminate unwanted anxiety, reaching into and removing problems at the deepest level without the need to dig deep into the recesses of the subconscious. This therapy can be used to conquer all manner of anxieties, including phobias, panic disorders, everyday stress, addictive urges, OCD and mild to severe trauma. It is used in psychiatry, psychology, general medical practice, hypnotherapy, NLP, and by social workers and teachers. However, the method is so simple that anyone can use it.

The therapy I am referring to is Thought Field Therapy – a revolutionary practice that is the single most effective way of taking the emotional sting out of your anxiety. It is a unique way of eliminating and managing anxiety and one that causes the minimum of distress. There may be a degree of upset – as it is necessary to think about the emotional problem – but essentially, for a few minutes of anxiety, you can get rid of life-long phobias, panic and anxieties.

History of Thought Field Therapy

Thought Field Therapy, or TFT, is a treatment for the rapid relief of all kinds of emotional and psychological distress. TFT takes the emotional charge out of a given situation. The memory stays but the intensity of the emotion diminishes or is completely eliminated.

The originator of TFT is Dr Roger Callahan, a clinical psychologist and an American pioneer of cognitive therapy and hypnotherapy. Having practiced for some 40 years, he was frustrated at how incredibly slow and ineffective traditional methods of psychotherapy were in facilitating change in individuals. Dr Callahan suffered from some severe anxieties himself – as a child, for instance, he was terrified of going through tunnels and of being in high-rise buildings.

He was passionate about finding a cure and explored many therapies, including Applied Kinesiology. It was his exploration that led to the development of TFT. Dr Callahan was treating a client called Mary for a water phobia that she had had since infancy. Although he had tried many different therapies with Mary, nothing seemed to make a significant difference. One day, when Dr Callahan was at his wits end, he heard Mary describe her phobia as 'feeling sick to her stomach'. He had learned about the meridian system and suggested that Mary tap under her eye (the stomach meridian). Miraculously the phobia disappeared.

Over time Dr Callahan continued his research and developed 'causal diagnosis', a method for determining the correct sequence of tapping the meridians to cure all manner of anxieties and psychological disturbances. These sequences are called algorithms. As I'm now a practising Thought Field therapist, Dr Callahan has very kindly given me permission to include several of his algorithms in this book. For in-depth knowledge I strongly recommend his own work, *Tapping the Healer Within*. For me, what is so wonderful about TFT is its simplicity. However, one must not forget the fact that these techniques have taken years to develop. Dr Callahan has indeed given us a gift.

Research on TFT

TFT may sound somewhat wacky, but the process is simple and incredibly effective. That effectiveness has been confirmed by a number of studies. In one, psychologists at Florida State University compared four different types of therapy, one of which was TFT. The study involved 156 people who had suffered a trauma or who had a severe phobia. The study, which evaluated the effectiveness of all four techniques using the SUD scale, found that whilst all four therapies were useful, TFT produced the greatest improvement and, most importantly, these improvements lasted over time. To this day, Dr Callahan's patient, Mary, has not suffered any recurrence of her water phobia.

The efficacy of TFT in treating post-traumatic stress disorder (PTSD) has also been shown. Since 1999, a number of TFT experts from the US, UK and Sweden have travelled to Kosovo to teach physicians how to use TFT with victims of PTSD. The physicians were treating people who had experienced unspeakable mental and physical abuse – trauma of the worst possible kind. Even in these circumstances, the success with TFT was exceptionally high and in 2002 TFT was recognized as a treatment of choice for trauma in Kosovo. (In the Appendix you will find a letter to Dr Callahan from the Chief of Staff of the medical battalion of K.P.C.).

It must be emphasized that taking the emotional charge out of a situation does not change the reality of the original event. You cannot change something that has actually happened. You can, however, take the emotional sting out of an event and change your emotional reaction to it, no matter how severe the trauma. If you have suffered any form of trauma in your life, TFT can enable you to become much stronger in the face of it.

THOUGHT FIELD THERAPY CHALLENGED THE NOTION THAT EMO-TIONAL SUFFERING IS HARD TO GET RID OF

TFT as Psychological First Aid

TFT, although originally designed to treat phobias, works effectively for a wide range of psychological and emotional states. It is an extremely powerful tool for treating general anxieties and panic attacks, as well as guilt, anger, jealousy and other anxiety-related conditions. My own personal success with TFT has been high. I find that simple phobias and anxieties are easily resolved but more complex cases take a bit longer. The most complex cases often require a practitioner to diagnose the meridian points that need to be addressed in order to deal with specific, individual problems. If symptoms do return this often indicates exposure to something else that may have affected the individual, for example, what Dr Callahan calls 'individual energy toxins'.

So what is Thought Field Therapy?

TFT includes elements from the quite diverse fields of clinical psychology, acupuncture, quantum physics and biology. It works on the basis that each thought has its own 'thought field'. This thought field contains information that forms the patterns of your thinking and hence shapes how you feel. When our feelings are negative or overly anxious, or events pop up that feel similar to a traumatic event in the past, the cause is in the thought field. It disrupts our energy circuitry and creates an imbalance. The thought field is related to the energy system of the body and tapping specific sequences of meridian points resolves the negative emotion. In the same way that we are unaware of our meridians, we are also not conscious of our thought field.

JUST BECAUSE YOU CAN'T SEE IT DOESN'T MEAN IT DOES NOT EXIST

By collapsing psychological blocks and disorders, TFT challenges the traditional thinking that all our memories are etched on our amygdala and are therefore indelible. TFT proves that the emotional content of our memories can be erased and therefore it is possible to take the negative emotional charge out of a painful experience.

Perturbations

According to Dr Callahan, negative emotions are caused by perturbations. These units of active information are the fundamental cause of all emotional suffering. Dr Callahan suggests that it is not the trauma itself that causes distress, but the information in the perturbation.

Experiences create perturbations and these perturbations are responsible for all the fundamental changes that are taking place within your
body when you are tuned in to that particular thought field. If you suffer from emotional malaise and ongoing stress and anxiety then there
are perturbations in your thought fields that need to be dealt with.

What does the Process Involve?

Tapping Your Energy Meridians

Perturbations are associated with specific energy meridians. Dr
Callahan discovered that by tuning into the thought field and tapping
into the energy meridians in a specific sequence (an algorithm) one
can deactivate the perturbation. These algorithms were identified by
Dr Callahan through the use of causal diagnosis. They are sets of steps
that have been tried and tested over the years – and you can use them
to tap out the disruption in your energy system and bring mental,
emotional and physical balance back to your body.

At the end of this chapter you will find an algorithm suitable for each
of the anxiety disorders featured in this book. However, before you can
tap out your anxiety, there are a number of processes that you need to
become familiar with.

In addition to using the appropriate algorithm to tap out the disruption in your energy system, we will be using a sequence developed
by Dr Callahan using ideas from Neuro-Linguistic Programming
(NLP). NLP is basically a method of changing our behaviour through
reprogramming how we think. NLP recognizes that the eyes are an
extension of the brain and that the movements of the eyes reflect how
and what we think. We move our eyes in certain directions to, for
instance, access memories, construct information, access our feelings
and to tune in to our own internal mental chatter.

In TFT, a sequence of eye movements is carried out whilst you tap a particular meridian and think about your anxiety. This contributes to the process of dismantling the negative emotion.

Humming and counting are also part of TFT treatment. Humming is thought to activate the right brain, while counting activates the left brain.

The Nine Gamut Sequence

The eye movements, tapping and humming are part of what is called the Nine Gamut Sequence, which supports the major tapping treatments that you will be using. In the nine gamut part of the procedure, the aforementioned eye processing, humming and counting are done whilst you simultaneously tap the gamut point – a spot on the back of the hand between the little and ring finger knuckles.

You may find it beneficial to try this before you do a complete algorithm. Begin by making a fist with your left hand. Now, viewing the back of the hand, take your index finger to the valley between the little finger and ring finger knuckles and move it down an inch towards your wrist. This is the gamut spot. Tap the gamut point and ensure that you keep your head still whilst doing the following procedure. Focus on the eye movements (if you cannot easily move your eyes do the sequence in your imagination).

★ close your eyes
★ open your eyes
★ look down to the left
★ now look down and to the right
★ take your eyes full circle in one direction
★ now do the same in the opposite direction
★ hum a few bars of any tune out loud
★ count aloud from one to five
★ hum that tune again

Floor to Ceiling Eye Roll

The eye roll is the final part of a TFT treatment. When you reach this stage you will have reduced your SUD score and your anxiety should have dissipated. The floor to ceiling eye roll promotes the relaxation response.

To do the eye roll you simply keep your head still and facing forward and start to tap the gamut point. Move your eyes down and now roll your eyes up towards the ceiling while continuing to tap the gamut point.

The SUD Scale

You have already been introduced to the SUD (subjective units of distress) scale in earlier chapters. This method of measuring your anxiety or discomfort involves simply tuning in to your feelings and measuring your anxiety level on a scale of one to ten (one being very little anxiety and ten maximum anxiety). When you come to do the appropriate algorithm, your responses should be written down so that you can measure your progress before and after treatment. It is important to be honest and accurate, as the only person you will be misleading is you. You are responsible for your own evaluation. You may find as you think about your anxiety that no feelings pop up. This could be because there are no perturbations present or, as is more likely, that you need to be exposed to the very thing you fear in order to experience the perturbation.

Tuning in to your Thought Field

It is vital that when you rate your anxiety, you focus on what you are feeling as you are experiencing the anxiety – not what you have experienced in the past or what you think you might feel in the future. You must associate into what you feel right at that moment. You may feel distressed or anxious as you tune in to the thought field but remind yourself that it is better to be distressed for a few minutes than for a lifetime. The major pay-off is that the anxiety that you are tuning into should disappear forever.

In order to collapse the perturbation in the thought field you need to focus on the anxiety that you want to get rid of. By doing this you will bring to the fore the relevant emotional disturbance. As you focus on how you feel right at that point, a cascade of chemical, mental, emotional and energetic changes will take place in your body. It's a bit like tuning into a radio station. You should then write down your SUD rating before you begin the appropriate algorithm.

The sequence of tapping can create a powerful shift in your body, deactivating perturbations and correcting the existing state of imbalance. At the end of the sequence of tapping take another SUD rating. This is an important way of measuring your progress. If your score has not gone down or has gone down slowly then this gives you further information. It could mean that you are not using the correct algorithm or you may be suffering from Psychological Reversal (more on this soon).

If the treatment has been successful, you will now be able to think about the subject without experiencing the negative emotional charge that was associated with it. When body and mind are in balance, your energy flows in uninterrupted patterns.

More Complex Cases

On occasions, the problem is not resolved immediately. This usually occurs because the thought that presents itself is only one aspect of the problem and there may be other thought fields involved. In such cases, further work has to be done and, similarly, you may find yourself using a different algorithm. These techniques are user-friendly. However, if your existing anxiety persists or comes back as strongly in intensity then I would suggest you find a TFT practitioner (see page 253) or seek the help of a health professional.

CASE STUDY The Apex Problem

A client called Monica came to see me in tears about a relationship that she had just finished. The man that she was dating worked overseas in the forces and she was worried not only about his safety but about being attached to someone who was away for such long periods of time. She decided to finish the relationship but was finding the process very painful. I gave her the TFT algorithm for love/pain. She found the process quite bizarre and afterwards insisted that she felt the same and no change had occurred. However, her SUD score had gone down from 8 to 2, she was no longer sobbing and colour had returned to her cheeks. When I bumped into her in the local sandwich shop later that day, she looked a completely different person and she confirmed that she felt fantastic. However, when I suggested that the treatment had worked she completely pooh-poohed the idea and said she didn't think it was the treatment at all.

The scenario described above often occurs with TFT, and is something Dr Callahan calls the Apex problem. It arises when someone uses TFT successfully but does not recognize that the treatment has been effective. The most common feedback that I receive is, 'I was distracted', 'my problem couldn't have been that big in the first place' or 'I couldn't have been *that* anxious'. With TFT, the treatment is so simple that people just don't seem to believe that a problem that they have had for so many years can disappear in moments. Many think that it will come back and they're simply experiencing momentary relief.

The Apex problem may also be a way for individuals to avoid having to confront the thought processes and challenges that may come as a result of clearing the perturbation. This can be a frequent occurrence with TFT and can therefore sabotage further treatment. Current thinking is that the Apex problem occurs because the left-brain is having difficulty rationalizing what has happened and creates its own irrelevant explanation.

TFT is not a Placebo

Many sceptics believe that TFT is a placebo. Placebos are thought to work because they mobilize an individual's expectation of getting better and hence activate their internal resources to make it happen. However, with TFT you do not have to believe in the process for it to work. In fact, many people have the treatment with the expectation that it won't work. They have negative expectations not positive ones, yet TFT still works for them.

Whilst being sceptical will not prevent the treatment working, it is important to recognize that it has worked. If your SUD levels are lower and your anxiety has dissipated then the treatment has worked. It is vital to acknowledge this so that all aspects of your anxiety can be worked on using the powerful techniques in this book. You must ensure, therefore, that you write down your SUD scores so you can reassure yourself of the difference. Lastly, test the effectiveness of the treatment by exposing yourself to the very thing that you previously feared. If you have lost the anxiety then TFT has worked!

Psychological Reversal

If you have treated yourself with TFT and you are still finding it difficult to eliminate anxiety then it is likely that you are suffering from Psychological Reversal, or PR. This is the most common block to successful treatment with TFT, or any other highly effective treatment. Psychological reversal is the term used in thought field therapy to describe a literal reversal of polarity. It describes a state of reversed energy direction in the body. If PR is present then you are unlikely to collapse a perturbation.

How would you know if you were suffering from psychological reversal? Well you may find that TFT has not worked at all, your SUD score has not gone down or that you are responding poorly to treatment. There are different variations of psychological reversal. Mini reversal can be related to a specific problem. As you think about the problem, your SUD score may drop from 8–9 to 6–7 instead of dropping to 2 or 1. Massive psychological reversal can be much more problematic and can affect your life more generally. If you suffer from massive psychological reversal it is likely that your attitude is negative and behaviours are self-sabotaging and defeating. PR can also recur after successful treatments. In many cases this is thought to be caused by exposure to energy toxins.

IF PR IS PRESENT YOU WILL NOT BE ABLE TO COLLAPSE THE PERTUR-BATION

Is psychological reversal treatable? The answer is yes, absolutely. There are a number of techniques that can be implemented to clear psychological reversal in its different variations. PR correction literally revives your system so that it returns to proper functioning. The PR correction technique that we will use in this book is tapping the karate point on the little finger side of the left or right hand.

It is important to emphasize that the following treatment is specific for psychological reversal and not the psychological problem. It is PR that is the problem, therefore it alone needs to be cleared in order for the treatment to work. After using the following techniques for PR, your SUD score – after repeating the treatment for the problem – should be considerably lower. This proves that the psychological reversal has been treated – clearing PR allows the perturbation in the thought field to be collapsed.

PR Correction Exercise – The Karate Point
The following exercise is for psychological reversal. Use it if your SUD score is going down slowly. You can also use it as a corrective procedure as often as you need it.

The PR correction spot, or karate point, is on the outer edge of either hand, between the wrists and the base of the little finger. Simply take two fingers and tap about 15 times. (For more information on psychological reversal please see *Stop the Nightmares of Trauma* by Dr Callahan.)

The Major Treatment Points

The different algorithms involve tapping the meridian points in a particular sequence. The twelve major meridian treatment points used in TFT are called the 'majors' of TFT. This term separates the main treatment from the other aspects of the treatment, for example tuning into the thought field, the nine gamut sequence, the PR treatment and the floor to ceiling eye roll. The majors are performed before and after the nine gamut sequence. The treatment points you need to be aware of to do the algorithms in this book are:

★ Eyebrow (EB): This point is at the beginning of the eyebrow just above the bridge of the nose.

★ Under the Eye (UE): This point is under the eye about an inch below the eyeball.

★ Collarbone (CB): This point is located an inch below the collarbone notch, a little to the right or left.

★ Under the Arm (A): This point is on the side of the body 4 inches under the armpit – level with the nipple for men and the middle of the bra strap for women.

★ Gamut spot: This is on the back of the hand between the little and ring finger knuckles, an inch down towards the wrist

★ Karate point: This is on the outer edge of either hand, between the wrists and the base of the little finger.

Each point is generally tapped about five times to stimulate the energy flow in the system. When you tap a meridian, tap firmly but not nearly so hard that you bruise yourself or cause pain.

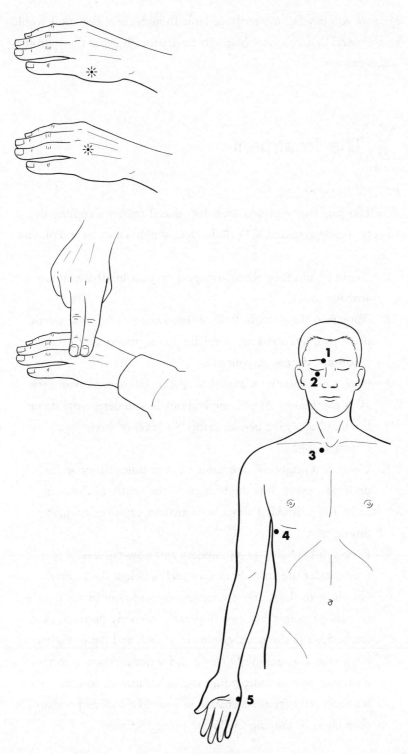

So now you have all the tools for basic thought field therapy. I would recommend that you now begin to treat yourself using the appropriate algorithm.

The Treatment

Algorithm One

The following algorithm is suitable for general anxiety, a combination of anxiety and depression, OCD, Body Dysmorphic Disorder and phobias.

1. Begin by thinking about an aspect of your life that you are anxious about.
2. Tune into the thought field of that anxiety – in other words, place your attention intentionally on an anxiety that produces emotional distress in your life.
3. Rate your anxiety on a level of one to 10 (one is no anxiety, 10 is maximum). As you think about this anxiety, write down the number which best describes the level of anxiety you are experiencing.
4. Using two fingers of one hand, tap five times about an inch under the eye, below the bottom of the centre of the bony orbit. Keep thinking about your anxiety. Tap firmly whilst tuning in.
5. Keep thinking about your anxiety and now tap solidly five times under the arm, about four inches below the armpit.
6. Continue to think about your anxiety and now firmly tap the collarbone point. Take two fingers to the bony protrusions at the bottom of the neck, go down an inch and tap to the right.
7. Now take a second SUD rating and write it down. If it has decreased two or more points then continue on to nine gamut sequence. If there is no change in your SUD score, perform PR correction by tapping the karate point 15 times.

8. Perform the nine gamut treatment. Tap the gamut point about three to five times per second and continue tapping whilst performing the following nine steps.

   ★ close the eyes
   ★ open the eyes
   ★ look down and left
   ★ open eyes down right
   ★ take eyes full circle in one direction
   ★ take eyes full circle in opposite direction
   ★ hum a few bars of your favourite tune
   ★ count from one to five
   ★ hum that tune

9. Now tap five times under the eye.

10. Tap five times under the arm.

11. Tap the collarbone five times.

12. Take another SUD reading and write it down. If it is down to one then do the eye roll. Keeping your head perfectly still, roll your eyes from the floor up towards the ceiling. If your SUD score has decreased but not as far as one then perform the PR correction exercise (see page 113), affirm that you will get over this anxiety and then repeat the treatment steps above.

Algorithm Two

This algorithm is specifically for depression.

1. Tune into the thought field by thinking about what you are depressed about.

2. On a scale of one to 10, rate your level of depression (one being no depression, 10 being very depressed). Write down your SUD rating.

3. Go to the gamut spot on the back of the hand between little and ring finger. Take two fingers and tap the gamut spot 30 times.

4. Tap the collarbone point at the centre of the collarbone where the two bones meet – go down an inch and move to the right

about one inch. Tap five times.

5. Take a second SUD reading. If it has decreased two or more points continue on to step 6. If there is no change, perform the PR correction exercise (see page 113) and then go through this process again.

6. Perform the nine gamut treatment. Go to the gamut spot at the back of the hand. Begin to tap the gamut spot with two fingers quickly 3–5 times per second and continue with the following treatment:

    ★ close the eyes
    ★ open the eyes
    ★ look down and left
    ★ open eyes and look down and right
    ★ fully circle your eyes in one direction
    ★ fully circle them in the other direction
    ★ hum a few bars of any tune aloud
    ★ count aloud from one to five
    ★ hum the tune again

7. Now tap the gamut spot 30 times.

8. Tap the collarbone point five times.

9. Take another SUD reading. If it is down more than one, go on to the last step. If it still has not decreased significantly perform the PR correction exercise and then repeat the steps above.

10. To finish off your treatment, hold your head level and move your eyes down. Then tap the gamut spot and roll your eyes up towards the ceiling.

Algorithm Three

This TFT treatment is suitable for social anxiety, panic attacks, PTSD and health anxiety.

1. Tune into the thoughts that bring on the feeling of anxiety.

2. Using the SUD scale think about how you feel right now on a level of one to 10 (1 is very little distress 10 is the worst

symptoms of panic). Write down the number.

3. Keep tuned into how you are feeling right now as you think about your distress and using two fingers of either hand, tap the spot at the eyebrow above the bridge of the nose. Tap this spot five times.

4. Keep tuned into your thought field and now tap about an inch under the eye five times.

5. Tap five times under the arm, about 4 inches under the armpit.

6. As you remain tuned into your area of anxiety, tap the collar-bone point – take two fingers of either hand to the collar-bone notch, move down an inch then move to the right one inch and tap five times.

7. Take second SUD reading and write it down. If it has decreased two or more points then go on to the nine gamut treatment below. However, if it has changed by only one point, do the PR correction exercise using the karate point.

8. Perform the nine gamut treatment. The gamut spot is at the side of the right or left hand between little finger and ring finger. Take your opposite hand to an inch below the knuckles of the ring finger. Begin to tap this spot with two fingers, continue tapping whilst going through the following nine steps:
   - ★ close the eyes
   - ★ open the eyes
   - ★ look down to the left
   - ★ point the eyes down and look down right
   - ★ circle the eyes in one direction right round
   - ★ circle the eyes in the opposite direction right round
   - ★ hum a few bars of your favourite tune
   - ★ count from one to five out loud
   - ★ hum the tune again

9. Now tap the eyebrow spot again five times.

10. Tap under the eye five times again.

11. Tap under the arm five times.

12. Tap the collarbone spot five times.
13. Take another SUD reading and write it down. If your score has now gone back down to one or less then do step 14. If your score has only gone down a little then perform the PR correction exercise (see page 113) and then repeat the treatment above.
14. To finish off, hold your head level and move your eyes down. Begin to tap the gamut point as you roll your eyes upwards.

How do you know if TFT treatment has worked?

The most obvious way is to go by what you feel. You may feel a sense of change, even if you can't put your finger on the exact amount of change, or you may have a sense of extreme wellbeing. Challenge yourself to try and bring the anxious feeling back into your body. If you can't, it has worked.

You can also observe the changes that are taking place in your physiology. You may, for instance, find your posture improving or the colour coming back into your cheeks as you breathe deeper and hence deliver more oxygen to your system.

Beliefs and Behaviours

The previous chapter illustrated that TFT is a powerful treatment that can eliminate unwanted anxiety from your life forever. However, the beauty of it lies not only in the fact that it can drastically reduce or eliminate emotional distress, but that it opens up the potential to further change your thinking. This is because beliefs that are fear-related can be changed or more easily challenged once the fear has been taken out of them. When the fear has gone, you open up the potential to believe something else instead.

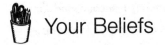 ## Your Beliefs

Challenging your beliefs is very important if you want to change your anxiety levels forever. In order to do this you need explore your current beliefs, behaviours and attitudes, and be open and willing to change the way you view your experience. You have a choice to make. Do what you have always done and you will get what you have always got. Believe what you have always believed and you could carry those beliefs with you into the future.

If your beliefs empower you then all well and good: if they disempower you they will have a negative effect on the way you live your life. It's amazing how people can continue to hold onto negative thinking patterns throughout their lives, despite the fact that they bring about self-destructive behaviour and anxiety. This anxiety is self-created and caused by a refusal to change.

CASE STUDY

On a trip to France with a group of friends and family, I was intrigued by the behaviour of our driver, who kept insisting that we were bound to get lost. He worried and obsessed about it and, not surprisingly, we did get lost. He then panicked and was so anxious he couldn't think clearly about where he was going. His panic increased as it got darker outside – this was even more proof of the doom that supposedly lay ahead for us.

Unfortunately his panic influenced everyone else in the car and although our 'navigator' had a very clear idea as to what to do, the driver's insistence that we were lost overrode any common sense whatsoever and created self-doubt in him, too. Having encouraged the driver to calm down by getting him to see that we were not in a life-threatening situation, I encouraged the other person to stick to his belief that he could get us to our destination. We soon arrived safely, although a little more tense and anxious than when we left home. When I suggested to the driver that his behaviour was not useful to him he shrugged his shoulders and said 'That's the way I am'.

Much anxiety is brought about by people refusing to change their existing beliefs. As a result, they often fail to take responsibility for their behaviour, blame others for their state of mind and create unnecessary anxiety for themselves. In truth, it would have been easy for the individual in the case study above to change his behaviour – if he had chosen to. It was his lack of belief in his own ability to find that destination that caused the problem – he had created a self-fulfilling prophecy. He chose stubbornly to stick to his belief, which made him panic and lose control.

In order to change negative behaviours that create a spiral of anxiety you need to explore what you believe. Beliefs are thoughts that shape and form in our mind. They are unconscious patterns that determine how you structure your experience – in other words, how you filter and format your experience of the world around you. Your thoughts become ideas and it is the emotional acceptance of these ideas that forms your beliefs. When you accept a belief as true it can become a generalization that frames your thinking. What you believe about something, whether positive or negative, will determine your attitude towards it.

Beliefs can remain constant or change over a lifetime. Core beliefs are generally formed in childhood, before our critical faculties have been developed and while we are too young to question them. Your beliefs are heavily influenced by your experiences. In the above case study, the driver's behaviour reflected his belief that unless you carefully plan and organize your life you are likely to fail and be out of control, with disastrous consequences. This had been drummed into him by a schoolmaster who had great influence over him.

Beliefs give meaning to your behaviour – 'I do this' because I believe this to be true. Beliefs can limit you or empower you and they can have a profound effect on your biology, as you automatically establish a reality out of what you believe to be true. I imagine our determined-to-be-lost driver lived his life very much in control but when a situation occurred to challenge his belief, he panicked. Beliefs are wrapped up in our expectations and this can influence your behaviour in such a way as to make what we expect to happen actually happen. Therefore, if you expect disasters to happen, you can often unwittingly encourage them to happen.

EXERCISE – WHAT ARE YOUR BELIEFS?

Write down two lists of current beliefs that you have – the first list should feature beliefs that empower you, while the second should be those that make you anxious and disempower you. Here are my two lists:

My empowering beliefs

1   You can do anything that you put your mind to, within reason.
2   We have all the resources within us to achieve our dreams.
3   I love my son.
4   My life gets better as I get older.
5   Exercise is excellent for stress and anxiety.

My disempowering beliefs

1   Relationships can be very trying.
2   I always forget people's names.
3   My cooking is awful.
4   I never have the time to do what I enjoy.

When you have written your lists, choose one belief from each list – the ones that stand out the most and you would most like to work on. First, think about the belief that empowers you. What is the evidence that this belief is true for you? How do you know that this belief is true? If you continue to have this belief in the future what will be the result for you? Think about how it enhances your life and could continue to do so even more in the future.

Now think about the belief that disempowers you. What is the evidence that this belief is true for you? What effect is this belief having on your life? Where did you learn this belief? You might want to do the Timeline exercise on page 79 to go back in time and explore the event or situation that may have created this belief (remember to do this exercise in a dissociated way). Now challenge the belief. How could this belief be wrong? Is this belief helpful or harmful and what will it cost you if you keep hold of it? Think five years into the future, 10 years, 20 years – what will happen if you continue to have this belief?

What would you rather believe instead? Write down your answer.

Begin to find experiences that back up your new belief. For beliefs to change you need to acquire new information.

Remember, beliefs are simply ideas and they can be changed if you wish. To change any beliefs you need to doubt their validity. You need to question them, challenge them, prove them wrong and focus on a belief that is more useful to you.

In the exercise above I wrote that my cooking is awful. I don't have time to cook – my life is too busy to spend time slaving over a hot stove. Plus I had an experience once when I decided to cook for friends and it was a disaster. For that I received a bit of a label – 'she cooks to kill'. However, I have recently proven that I can cook well – when I put my mind to it. It is no longer true that my cooking is lousy. I would rather believe that I can cook just as well as anyone else and, when I put my mind to it, I cook very well.

Develop a statement of what you would rather believe instead. Mine is now – I know that I am a great cook and I am even better when I have the time for it.

EXERCISE – PIN DOWN YOUR REASONS

If you are finding it difficult to believe your preferred belief, ask yourself what purpose there is in continuing to have the old, limiting belief. Often such beliefs have a very powerful purpose, in that they sustain safety behaviours that you have developed – for example, 'it keeps me safe' or 'helps me fit in with others'.

My reason for believing that I was an awful cook was because it let me off the hook if I did concoct a disaster. Also, I would-n't get asked to do it very often and could get on with my work instead.

Beliefs and your Behaviour

Beliefs result in behaviour that is either positive or negative. Your behaviour is what you express externally as a result of inner dialogue you have with yourself, and the beliefs that you hold. All behaviours are learned. We develop them ourselves or we model ourselves on others. How many times have you found yourself behaving in a way that your parents or grandparents do? Behaviours that are repeated become habitual through that repetition.

The first step towards change is to look at your behaviour, particularly when it creates anxiety. Don't judge yourself for behaving in a particular way, simply ask yourself if it is useful to you or not. Think about the consequences of your behaviour if you keep on doing it.

Behind every behaviour is the intention to achieve something that is of value to you. There is always a higher purpose. Now that may sound strange, especially if you think of your behaviour as negative or destructive, but whether your behaviour is empowering or limiting the intention behind it is positive. How do you uncover that higher purpose? You simply ask yourself the question 'what does this behaviour do for me?' Wait for the answer (write it down) then ask the question again of whatever answer comes up. The following example – of some-one who comfort eats – illustrates what I mean.

What does comfort eating do for me?

It makes me less stressed

What does feeling less stressed do for me?

It makes me relax more

What does relaxing do for me?

It makes me feel lighter and enjoy life more

Once you know the intention that lies behind the behaviour you wish to change, you can begin to explore other ways of achieving the desired outcome. The following exercise will help you do just that.

EXERCISE – REFRAMING

1 *Think of behaviour that makes you anxious and that you want to change.*

2 *Ask yourself what the positive intention of this behaviour is for you. Ask yourself this question until you get to that higher purpose.*

3 *Inside yourself there is a part of you that is able to generate new behaviours easily and effortlessly. Ask this part to generate two new behaviours that will satisfy that positive intention. Write them down.*

4 *Ask yourself 'does any part of me object to performing these new behaviours?' If there are any parts that object, find out the intention behind this and go through the process again.*

5 *Once you feel that all of you is in agreement, imagine a movie screen in your head, with you in the picture practising your new behaviours. See how you will be different and notice how these changes affect your state.*

6 *Think of the different areas of your life where you can now practice these new behaviours.*

Mixed Behaviours

One of the greatest causes of anxiety is having mixed feelings about something. The internal strife that this can cause makes us feel that we are being pulled in different directions and are incapable of making a decision. Often when this happens, the conflict is reflected in our behaviour. We may, for example, say yes to something whilst our head is busily shaking from side to side and not up and down. In NLP this is called incongruence. This means that your external behaviour does not match your internal processing. Your mouth may be saying one thing, but your heart and body language another.

Although the subconscious mind is a whole mechanism, sometimes we develop 'parts' – and this can result in conflict in the mind. These parts have been described as non-integrated parts of the whole. They are often like minor personalities and seem to have an intelligence and beliefs or values system of their own. These parts of your character are born as a result of emotional events that have affected your thinking. The slow drip of life's events can also create parts, as we develop different strategies or 'personalities' to cope with the various challenges of life.

When you are congruent, both mind and body are in complete harmony and agreement with each other – you feel whole. It is common to feel congruent in some areas of life and incongruent in others. Usually, people are more successful and calm in the areas where they are congruent. In contrast, areas of incongruence create anxiety.

EXERCISE – HOW CONGRUENT ARE YOU?

Explore your own experience. Think of the areas in your life that you are anxious about. Are you congruent in your behaviour? Do you back up positive language patterns with positive body language? Is your conscious and unconscious willpower in harmony or are you incongruent i.e. do you say one thing while your body language says another? Think about the different states of mind that the two bring. Are you aware of parts of yourself in conflict? Which part creates more anxiety for you?

If you are incongruent – and most of us are in some area of our lives – the following exercise is a very good way of uncovering what lies behind the conflict. The objective of the exercise is to explore two or more parts that are not in agreement and hence understand their higher functions and get them to begin to work together.

EXERCISE – RECONCILING PARTS

Think of an area of your life where you have mixed feelings. Imagine these conflicting parts as actors on a stage and put one on each hand. You may want to give them names and a description – are they male or female? Now pay attention to each part and find out about them. Ask each part to reveal its highest intention, that which is most important for them to achieve. After each answer, keep asking this question until they discover what they both ultimately want. You may find that it is the same thing, such as wholeness, happiness, joy, freedom, safety or security. Have both parts recognize they were once part of a larger whole. Ask each part if they are prepared to work with the other and, if there is any resistance, find out what that might be. Ask each part to come up with different ways of working together, so that they can reach their shared goal more easily.

Now allow these parts to integrate in their own way. You may find that your hands want to come together automatically.

If you experience resistance then create a third part with the combined resources of each part. Place this third part between both parts and now allow them to integrate.

CASE STUDY

Kevin, a 35-year-old businessman, was having problems making career decisions. He was in a job where he felt uninspired and although he wanted to move on, a part of him was resisting. This conflict caused him great anxiety and he developed depression as a result.

We did the reconciling parts exercise above and explored what was behind the part of him that was putting up resistance. He heard the voice of his father in this part, saying things like you should do this, you should do that or you have failed. This part had a fear of failure. I did the Timeline exercise to uncover the origin of this fear and Kevin went back to being a three-year-old and being corrected by his father. He was able to let go of the fear as he explored the event from an adult's point of view and challenge the belief that he was holding. Once we cleared the origins of the belief we were able to find that both parts had the same purpose and they were able to integrate to enable him to feel more whole.

Behaviour is not Identity

Lastly, it is important to understand that all behaviour is learned behaviour and your behaviour is not who you are. Often we tend to be intolerant of individuals or judge them, when really it is their behaviour that needs to be addressed and not who they are. This is very common when dealing with children. When they acquire or perform behaviours that are not useful, parents often make them feel bad or chip away at their confidence by making comments such as 'you are a bad girl' or 'you stupid boy'. But more often it is the child's behaviour that need addressing, not the character of the child. If you accept someone for who they are and separate them from their behaviour this creates less friction and anxiety and makes good relationships easier.

By separating the individual and how they behave, you also make it easier for them to discard behaviour that is not useful to them. And, of course, this applies to how you view your own behaviour, too. Don't make the mistake of thinking your behaviour is 'who you are'. It isn't, it's simply something you've acquired and hence it's something you can choose to discard.

Power Tool 2 – Self–Hypnosis

By now you should have taken the emotional charge out of your anxieties through TFT. In so doing you will have made it easier to change your beliefs and behaviour – because the more open and flexible you can be, the more choices you have.

Having looked at the role of the parasympathetic system in bringing the body back into balance, we'll now examine how to relax and reprogram your thinking through self-hypnosis. In TFT you tune into the body's thought field. With self-hypnosis you tune in to your internal world through the power of suggestion. When you do this, you can actually reprogram your thinking – you can guide and direct your mind to bring about the most amazing transformational changes in your anxiety levels and indeed your life.

An anxious mind cannot exist within a relaxed body
EDMUND JACOBSON

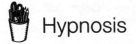 ## Hypnosis

The word hypnosis is derived from the Greek word for sleep. Hypnosis is a powerful, natural phenomenon that has been around for thousands of years and is, perhaps, as old as mankind. The hypnotic state has been given a number of different names at different times and in different cultures: mesmerism, voodoo, the reverie state, animal magnetism, trance … It is, in fact, a very similar state to meditation, which is a state of contemplation or reflection. Unfortunately, many misconceptions about hypnosis persist even today, in part as a result of unfounded sensationalist theories and stage hypnosis. At the forefront of those misconceptions is the idea that a hypnotist can take control of your mind.

Hypnosis and Mind Control

There are many things that can exert a degree of influence over us –
as children it's parents, teachers and society in general, while as adults
it's usually anything from television to drink and drugs. However, it is
not possible for a hypnotist to control your mind.

As adults, we have belief systems that we adhere to and anything that
does not conform to that system we reject. This is why, in hypnotherapy, client and practitioner work together to reprogram the individual's
thought processes. A hypnotherapist cannot put thoughts and suggestions into someone's head if that person does not want them. We have
a free will. If anything inappropriate is suggested, the critical faculties
of the conscious mind will kick in and the individual will bring themselves out of hypnosis.

With self-hypnosis – which is what you will be mostly using in this
book – you take complete charge of your own programming and
thought patterns. You can create your own suggestions and visualizations for absolutely any area of life through the use of scripts (more on
this later). With self-hypnosis you take full responsibility for your
change. And it works – it has for hundreds of thousands of people and
it will for you, too.

Is Hypnosis Part of the Occult?

Absolutely not! In fact, it can be likened to prayer. Guess what prayer
is – making repeated suggestions whilst in a contemplative frame of
mind. For centuries, many different religions have encouraged prayer
or meditation. Those that banned it generally did so out of a fear that
it would somehow negate the need for organized religion. Today hypnosis is endorsed by most of the major religions.

For those who are religious, hypnosis can intensify faith. When you
go into hypnosis, you bring about the same higher states of mind that

you achieve in meditation. In this state the irrelevant clutter that clogs the mind is brushed aside, allowing you to become more in tune with your faith.

The Practice of Hypnosis Today

Hypnosis can be used in many different areas of life. In the 1950s both the American Medical Association (AMA) and British Medical Association (BMA) recognized hypnosis as a powerful aid to the medical world. Today it is used for everything from anxiety disorders and stress management, to dentistry, childbirth and other areas where pain control is needed. It has also been proven that the subconscious mind can help the body develop a greater resistance to infection and improve recovery time. It is also very effective in many other areas of life – smoking cessation, weight management, sports performance and personal development are just a few.

The success of hypnotherapy very much depends on the competence of the practitioner. Hypnosis, however, is not only the preserve of the professional hypnotherapist – everybody can use it in a very simple way.

HYPNOSIS CAN HELP YOU HARNESS YOUR AMAZING RESOURCES AND GUIDE YOU TO MORE RESOURCEFUL STATES OF MIND

How Does Hypnosis Work?

There are four primary brain wave patterns – beta, alpha, theta and delta. We spend most of our working time in the beta state, where we are alert and capable of critical thought. We frequently switch from this to the alpha state, although we are often not aware of it. The alpha state is a state of serenity, relaxation and detached concentration. We are in the theta state at least twice a day, usually in the morning just as we awaken, or when we are on the brink of sleep. This is the state in which people are at their most creative, producing ideas and solutions to problems. The theta state also activates the relaxation response in the body, causing the muscles to relax and the heart rate and breathing to slow down and work at their natural rhythms. The delta state comes only with deep sleep. In this state we process information through our dreams. It is a period of rejuvenation and cell renewal.

The most useful states for self-hypnosis are alpha and theta. When both body and mind come together in these states you have a relaxed and calm mind. It is then more open to the suggestions you make.

What is Self-Hypnosis?

Quite simply, self-hypnosis is the ability of the individual to place themselves in a state of hypnosis. In the hypnotic state, the conscious mind recedes and the subconscious mind comes to the fore. To achieve this state it helps to become completely relaxed in both mind and body – only then can you communicate directly with your unconscious mind.

Can Anyone do Self-hypnosis

Yes, although I do not recommend you do it under the influence of drugs or alcohol or if you have a severe mental disorder. There are different levels of hypnosis, from light trance to deeper levels, but it is possible for anyone to reach these stages through the power of suggestion. Relaxation is fundamental to the process of self-hypnosis in this book and it is a skill that can be learned just like any other.

What are the Benefits of Self-hypnosis?

★ It makes problem solving easier. When the mind is free of clutter you can focus on what you really want.

★ It increases creativity. When we quieten the conscious mind and allow the subconscious to become dominant, our inherent creativity rises to the surface, too.

★ The mind accepts suggestions and visualizations more readily because it is not operating under the strictures of the conscious mind.

★ At a mental and emotional level, it can release emotional blockages and calm the mind.

★ The relaxation inherent in hypnosis regenerates and rejuvenates all the cells in your body, which can increase your energy and vitality.

Relaxation is fundamental to the process of hypnosis, but it is a skill that can be learned just like any other. To relax means making a conscious decision to let go and enter into a world you may never have experienced before. Once there you can take complete control of your internal processing – you can work through any challenges that you may face and focus on your goals for the future, finding the ways and means to achieve them.

How Long should I Stay in Hypnosis?

With the techniques we are using it may take a little time and practise to achieve hypnosis. Give yourself 15 to 30 minutes for the whole procedure. After a bit of practise, and with the techniques given, you will be able to put yourself in hypnosis within minutes and then make the changes that are needed. This should take 10 to 15 minutes.

However, you can stay in hypnosis for as long as you like and simply come out of it when you are ready.

Beliefs and Expectations of Hypnosis

The success of hypnosis relies completely on your beliefs and expectations. Often people expect hypnosis to be something that it is not and when they come out of it they don't believe that they have been hypnotized. If you believe hypnosis won't work then it won't. If you want it to work it will work. It may take a little bit of practice but as long as your mind is open and the desire is there you will achieve a level of hypnosis.

Essentially you are responding to the power of suggestion, irrespective of whether those suggestions are coming from you or somebody else. If you follow the process in an open way, believe it will work and expect it to work then it will.

⚘ Hypnosis – the Gateway to the Unconscious

There are literally thousands of ways to induce hypnosis. Suggestion is at the heart of the matter, so in this practical section we will look at how to use suggestion in a way that will produce a hypnotic response. It is important to note that the subconscious mind is very literal in its interpretation so it is important to use language correctly. Although we will be using the spoken word to induce hypnosis and make changes where necessary, language does not come in words alone, it comes in pictures, sensations and feelings. The following guidelines therefore offer advice for using all of your senses, not just the spoken word.

Guidelines for Self-hypnosis

★ Be Positive

Talk yourself into hypnosis by using positive language to relax your body and mind. Positive suggestions will make you feel less anxious and more empowered and relaxed. The subconscious is the seat of the emotions and the more you suggest calm, relaxed emotional states the more your body will respond. When in hypnosis, use powerful positive emotional descriptions to achieve your desired state. Begin by changing the negative words that you may currently use to describe your anxiety and use positive words instead. Focus on what you wish to achieve and focus on the positive good that will come from achieving a more resourceful state of mind. The subconscious mind is goal orientated so focus on what you want rather than what you don't want. Create positive images of your goal. Imagine how you want to feel using positive words – for example, 'I am no longer anxious' will make you focus on the very thing you don't want. It would be better to say 'I am calmer every day'. Instead of 'I won't be scared at my interview' use 'I look forward to my job interview'. See yourself as you wish to be. Hear yourself as you wish to be heard. Feel as you wish to feel.

★ Be Specific

Ensure your language is specific about what you wish to achieve. If you want to be relaxed then take yourself through a physiological relaxation and use appropriate language to induce relaxation. If it is to mentally cleanse your mind then use suggestions to free the mind of all clutter. Cover every detail of the desired change that you want to make and take the time to make use of some good descriptive words. For example, if your goal is to be calm and relaxed in interviews you could add even more positive energy by saying 'I look forward to my interview in a calm and a relaxed way' or 'I am thrilled to have the opportunity to attend this interview and I am calm and relaxed throughout'. Use vibrant, energetic and persuasive words such as easily, effortless, bright, thrilling, amazing. You can also be specific about time so you could, for example, say 'At 11.45, just before the interview, I become even more calm, relaxed and centred'.

Make sure your suggestions are about you and not others. You cannot change others. However, you can change yourself, which then often facilitates change in others. So it is not advisable to say 'when I walk into the interview everybody will admire me'. Use words that target your outcome clearly and precisely.

★ Be Realistic

An essential part of self-hypnosis is to work within your belief system. Hence, you need to use suggestions that are realistic and achievable and that you know your subconscious will respond to. A pre-requisite of successful change is being realistic about what is achievable. This is often where people go astray. If you set your standards too high, you are likely to give up. I had a client who set herself a target of losing a considerable amount of weight in a certain amount of time. In order to do this she told herself that she would exercise every day, however she lost faith and gave up fairly quickly when she discovered she couldn't exercise every day and therefore lose the weight as quickly as she wanted. She needed to change her strategy and her language to be successful. She could commit to three times a week so we changed her suggestion to 'As I exercise consistently I am getting closer and closer to achieving my goal weight'.

★ Be Repetitive

The subconscious mind loves repetition. When you repeat a suggestion you are giving it your attention, and the more you strengthen the suggestion the more likely it is to become real. You can either repeat exactly the same suggestion or reword it. As you take yourself into hypnosis, for example, you could say 'every nerve, muscle, cell in my body relaxes' or 'the whole of my body relaxes from the top of my head to the tip of my toes'.

Repeat your affirmations to yourself throughout the day as well as during hypnosis and whenever you need reminding. And repeat the words even if you feel resistance. (After all if you really did believe you were calm you wouldn't have to say it.) Saying the words, repeating the words and acting as if they were true will make them true.

★ Be in the Present

Your subconscious mind responds best to language in the present tense. It will comply with whatever suggestions it is given and if you keep saying 'I am no longer as nervous as I was last week' your point of focus will be last week's nervousness and you're likely to just feel nervous again. If you want to set a target for the future when under hypnosis you must still talk to yourself in the present tense and give the achievement of that goal a specific time frame – for instance, 'every day I am working towards becoming calm and relaxed'. Speaking in the present tense avoids confusion.

★ Be Active

Ensure you focus your language on action rather than ability. You subconsciously will respond better. So, instead of saying 'I know I have the ability to be calm and relaxed', say 'I am becoming more and more calm and relaxed. I am in control of my life'.

★ Set a Time Limit

Set a specific time by which you will have successfully achieved your target and then take yourself through the process that is needed to get you there – for example, when will be appropriate for you to have stopped smoking completely? How long will it take to begin to feel calmer and more confident about yourself? How long will it take for you to make the perfect presentation? How long will it take for you to see the benefits of believing in yourself more? This will give you markers to work towards and a greater awareness of the process of getting to where you want to go.

★ Be Simple

To induce hypnosis and communicate effectively with the subconscious mind it is vital to use language that is simple. The subconscious mind is like a 10-year-old child – it will respond better to simple suggestions than complex ones. Complicated language is likely to be less effective.

Further Steps Towards Self-hypnosis

Your Primary Representational System

Each of us makes sense of our world in a different way. We take in information from the world around us through our senses – what we see, hear, feel, smell and taste – and then recreate and represent what we experience in the world in our own minds. In NLP, the sensory system is referred to as the representational system. Most of us tend to think in pictures, sounds and sensations, hence we rely on our visual, auditory or kinaesthetic senses. However, while we all use each of these representational systems, we tend to favour one over the rest. Knowing which one you favour is very useful for self-hypnosis because it means you can use the most appropriate and effective representation system to enhance your affirmations, visualizations and scripts.

To establish your dominant representational system tick which of the following statements are most true to you.

★ I mostly think in pictures (V)
★ I think in sounds (A)
★ I seem to think according to how I feel (K)
★ It is mostly what I see either externally or internally that triggers anxiety (V)
★ I become anxious in response to my internal chatter (A)
★ I communicate my anxiety by the feelings that I share (K)
★ The decisions that I make are heavily influenced by what I see (V)
★ I make decisions when something sounds right (A)
★ My decisions are determined by my gut feeling (K)
★ I must see things to understand them (V)
★ I learn by listening (A)
★ I learn by doing (K)

V = visual, A = auditory, K = kinaesthetic

Using Language

You can also establish what representational system you use by listening to the sort of language you use.

Visual

Predominately visual people will use lots of 'visual' words such as look, see, picture, view, clear, image, appear, show, focused, crystal, hazy. Typical phrases they may use include things like I'm much clearer now, get an eyeful of that, in light of, don't make a scene, take a peek … and so on.

Auditory

People who are predominantly auditory use lots of words such as hear, sound, tone, talk, tune, listen, feedback, silence, harmonize, resonate. Typical phrases that they use would be: that sounds good to me, I hear you loud and clear, clear as a bell, describe that in detail …

Kinaesthetic

People who use a predominantly kinaesthetic system will use lots of 'feeling' language, for example words like grasp, handle, calm, touch, solid, sensation, hard, soft etc. Phrases typical of the kinaesthetic person would be something along the lines of: I can handle that, control yourself, you're a smooth operator, pain in the neck/butt, get a load of this …

Eye Accessing Cues

Yet another way to establish how you process information is to think about how you use your eyes. As we discovered in chapter 5, the eyes reflect what is going on in the brain. When an individual is visualizing, the eyes go up and either to the left or right or straight ahead; when they're hearing something, the eyes go to the right or left side in line with the ears; when they're thinking about their feelings, the eyes go down and right; and when they're having a conversation with themselves, they go down and left.

**EXERCISE – GUESS THE
REPRESENTATIONAL SYSTEM**

*You can do this exercise alone or with a friend. Let your friend
talk about their favourite subject for two or three minutes and
see if you can decipher what representation system they are
using. Listen to the language that is predominately used and
watch how the eyes move. To do the exercise alone, simply talk
about your favourite subject without trying to exert too much
control over what you say and then think about your choice
of words.*

Considerations for Different Representational Systems

The following information is important, irrespective of your dominant
representational systems. Obviously particular sections will resonate
more with those who have that dominant representation system, but
please read through all the information on the senses as they can all
play a part in making self-hypnosis more effective.

Your Auditory Senses

If you are making your own tapes or CDs for the purposes of self-
hypnosis, the sound of your own voice will influence how you
respond – particularly if you are predominately auditory. Don't try to
use what you think is a hypnotic tone – it will only sound false. With
self-hypnosis it is better to speak normally and clearly in a tone that
generates warmth and receptiveness. The tone of your voice should
make you want to respond to what you say. You may want to put
emphasis on words to enhance their effect but resist any temptation to
use unnatural tones and instead speak in a warm, clear voice that is
compelling. You may also want to consider using gentle music in the
background or the sounds of the sea or nature. For many this enhances
relaxation.

EXERCISE – FIND YOUR VOICE

Practise reading from a book or a script using a voice that is warm and compelling. You may want to practise this by recording and listening to your voice a few times. Allow yourself to settle on the voice that sounds most natural to you. When you are recording a tape for yourself, use 'you' as if you were talking to someone else – then when you play the tape back you will be talking to yourself. However, when you're simply repeating a script, and not recording it, use 'I'.

You may also want to use distinctly 'auditory' language to induce self-hypnosis and to create scripts and statements for change. You may find the following example useful:

▼ EXAMPLE OF AUDITORY SUGGESTION ▼

As you hear the sound of my voice you relax more and more. Any other sounds just fade into the distance as you now only pay attention to the sound of my voice taking you deeper and deeper into relaxation. As you now pay attention to all your bodily sensations – the beating of your heart, the rhythm of your breath – all mental chatter just seems to fade away.

Your Visual Sense

As I mentioned before, language does not just occur in the form of words. Language is both verbal and non-verbal and part of that non-verbal communication is vision. In fact, it is thought that words make up a small amount of our 'language'. We possibly rely on vision more than any of the other senses to make sense of the world around us.

Although you may not be aware of it, we think naturally in images all the time. The images that you create may be positive or negative, depending on what you are thinking at the time but, whichever it is, the subconscious mind will literally work like a robot to obey the instructions it is being given. So if you make fearful, anxious pictures then your subconscious will get the message to create fearful, anxious biology.

What your mind sees your body will respond to physically. Your attitude can create changes in the brain through the nervous system and the glandular system, triggering the production of hormones such as stress hormones and creating or deepening neural pathways. If you recall, the subconscious mind is also responsible for your imagination and it cannot tell the difference between a real and an imaginary experience. That may sound like a sweeping statement but it is true. If you've ever experienced jumping or jerking yourself awake when you have had a frightening dream then you have already experienced this. This was your body responding to those dreams as if they were real. Are you still in doubt? Try the following exercise.

EXERCISE – USE YOUR IMAGINATION

Close your eyes and imagine a lemon – a nice juicy lemon. See the yellow colour and waxy texture of that lemon. Imagine the lemon cut in half with all the juices spilling out. Now imagine biting into that lemon.

What did you notice? Some of you would have noticed tangy sensations; some would have salivated as you saw the juiciness of that lemon in your mind's eye. But you may also have noticed how your mind responded to the picture that you gave it. Often our brain creates pictures in response to our perceived or actual threats and challenges. When this happens the body responds as if each threat were real.

THE SUBCONSCIOUS MIND CANNOT TELL THE DIFFERENCE BETWEEN A REAL AND AN IMAGINERY EXPERIENCE

Now that you know you have a very real physiological response to the directions you give yourself, you can use your imagination to get your body to respond to the suggestions that you give it. The more relaxed you imagine yourself to be, the more relaxed you will become. For a predominately visual person, the most effective strategy is to use visual words to induce hypnosis and to visualize the process of deepening relaxation as you go through it. You may find the following example of how to intensify relaxation useful:

▼ EXAMPLE OF VISUALIZATION FOR ▼
DEEPENING RELAXATION

As you go inside your body, see all your internal systems slowing down and working at their natural place, working at their natural rhythm. See the tension leaving your body as you go deeper. See yourself looking calm and completely relaxed. See the waves of relaxation flowing over you and through you. See yourself as you wish to be – relaxed, calm, at ease within yourself.

You can also use your visual skills for goal-setting and imagining the changes that you want to take place (see Visualization page 177).

Your Kinaesthetic Sense

Kinaesthetic sensations relate to our emotions and bodily sensations such as balance, temperature and muscle tension. Although we may be aware of how we feel, we also need to recognize that often such feelings are produced in response to our internal dialogue and the visual images that we create in our mind. Kinaesthetic sensations also occur in association with memories – pleasant memories bring about pleasant feelings; unpleasant memories evoke unpleasant feelings. We can also induce kinaesthetic sensations through using our imagination.

Using kinaesthetic language for self-hypnosis will help you to focus on how you feel and wish to feel during hypnosis. The following example illustrates the sort of language that is useful:

▼　EXAMPLE OF KINAESTHETIC SUGGESTION　▼

With every breath I take I feel even more relaxed and at ease. Every time I think of my presentation [or whatever the cause of anxiety is], I simply take a deep breath and feel more relaxed and calm.

We will also use the breath and suggestions to deepen and change bodily sensations during the state of hypnosis. Good bodily awareness is an important tool for counteracting anxiety.

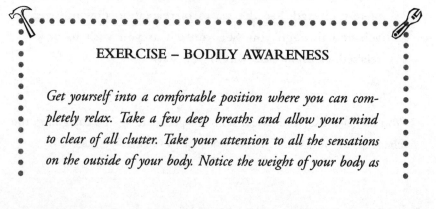

EXERCISE – BODILY AWARENESS

Get yourself into a comfortable position where you can completely relax. Take a few deep breaths and allow your mind to clear of all clutter. Take your attention to all the sensations on the outside of your body. Notice the weight of your body as you sit or lie down. Take your awareness to your clothing and notice how that clothing feels against your body. Now notice your body temperature – is it warm or cool? Take your attention to all the muscles in your body – are they tense or relaxed? Start at the head and work your way down, noticing how your body feels. Be aware of tightness, tension, pressure, tingling sensations ... Lastly, take your awareness to the breath – how is your breathing?

How can you use all of this information for self-hypnosis? When you have worked out your dominant representational system you can use it to make hypnosis more personal and more effective for you. You can also explore your weaker senses and make them stronger. For example, if you are mainly visual, are you aware of that quiet little voice that is making you anxious? Tune in and listen to what it is saying and you will be able to intervene and make a change if the dialogue is not useful. Similarly, a kinaesthetic person can draw their attention away from their feelings and into their visual or auditory senses to make greater sense of them.

Some Practicalities

Environment

Before we move onto the hypnotic induction, it is important to set up the right environment in which to practise. Your environment affects your state and your state will affect your performance. The correct environment for self-hypnosis is one where you cannot be disturbed, there is minimum noise, the surroundings are visually pleasing, and where you feel warm and comfortable. Warmth is important because the body becomes cooler as your muscles relax. If it is a warm day, ensure the room is well ventilated.

Timing

The time of day you choose to practise is down to you, although first thing in the morning or last thing at night is generally best as this is when the mind is more likely to be in a state conducive to relaxation.

Position

The most comfortable positions in which to relax are lying down and sitting with your back against a chair. The latter is probably best if you are prone to nodding off. If you are sitting make sure that your feet are on the floor. You can use cushions to make yourself more comfortable. You may also use cushions under your knees if you have a bad back and are lying down.

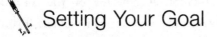 ## Setting Your Goal

I have mentioned a number of times that the subconscious mind is goal orientated and will work towards the goals that you give it, be they positive or negative. So one way of improving your anxiety levels is to take control of the goals that you set yourself. If you give your subconscious mind more positive points of focus, you will achieve greater wellbeing.

If you keep focusing on what you don't want, it's quite likely that you may get it – or go through high levels of anxiety in order to avoid it. Some people don't set goals for fear of failure; others fear success or, more commonly, the feedback that it may entail. If this applies to you, you need to use the TFT algorithm on page 116 to eliminate these fears. You then need to explore your beliefs and begin to think about how you can change your thinking.

YOU GET WHAT YOU FOCUS ON

The following NLP exercise is a simple but effective way of setting your outcome for the future. I suggest you use it for thinking about what you most want to achieve. Your goals may be small or large but the more specific you can be about what you want, the more likely you are to get it.

EXERCISE – CHOOSE YOUR OUTCOME

Ask yourself 'what do I want to achieve from Anxiety Toolbox?' The more specific and clear your answer, the more likely you are to get it. For example, someone with OCD may say 'I want to be able to leave my house every day in a calm way, knowing that I have turned everything off.' Other outcomes could be, 'Every time I fly I want to enjoy the experience'.

Focus on the Benefits
Once you know what you want, the next question to ask yourself is 'If I were to get what I wanted what would that do for me?' Think about the benefits that you will achieve from reaching your goal. Write down the first answer that comes into your head. Then look at that answer and ask yourself 'and what will that do for me?' Keep on asking yourself that question until you get some benefit at a much higher level, for example:

If I were able to leave my house knowing that I have turned everything off I would feel relieved.
If I were relieved I would relax more.
If I were to relax more I would feel more comfortable about myself.
If I were to feel more comfortable about myself I would feel more normal.
If I were to feel more normal I would like myself more.
If I liked myself more I would be at peace.

Use Your Senses

The next question to ask yourself is 'How will I know that I have achieved this outcome?' What would you see, hear and feel if you were to achieve it? The objective is to get your brain working in a positive way for you by getting your senses to construct a clear, sensory description of the desired outcome. The person with OCD, for example, may conjure up the following scene:

I see myself turning off everything just once. Then I see myself checking just once and then happily leaving my house and going about my day. I hear me telling myself this is now turned off, that is turned off and my gut feeling would be trust that I have done these things. I feel much later lighter, happier and more relaxed.

Resources and Self-Maintenance

The next question to ask yourself is 'If I were to achieve this outcome would I be able to maintain it and what resources do I need to maintain it?' Consistency is vital – you need to keep reminding yourself of the benefits that you are working towards and finding ways to measure your progress and ensure that you keep going. Your answer to the above question should therefore be along the lines of:

Yes I can maintain this. I will make time and put into practise my new behaviours and thinking. I will know that I am getting there by doing the behaviours that I need to do and feeling much calmer about doing them.

In What Context Do You Want This Outcome?

The next questions will then be 'in what context would you want this outcome? When do you want it? When don't you want it? With whom do you want it and with whom don't you want it?' For our OCD sufferer, the answer might be:

I want this mainly at home but also at the office. As I am the last to leave, it is down to me to lock up and make sure all the computers are switched off.

Ecology

When you set a goal you need to be sure that it accommodates all aspects of life that are important to you. In other words, you need to be aware of the overall consequences of your change. In NLP this is called an ecology check – because it means looking at our personal ecology i.e. how the outcome will affect all the interrelated aspects of our life.

You therefore need to ask 'what is the ecology of this outcome for me? Is it worth it? Is it worth the time, money and effort it will take to achieve it? How will others be affected as a result of my achieving this outcome?'

Again, using our OCD sufferer as an example, the answer may be:

Others will benefit enormously. I will arrive at work much calmer. Others will be able to relax around me and be less anxious, too. I will be a much nicer person. I will have so much more time for other things. It is absolutely worth doing whatever I have to do to achieve this.

What is the next step from here?

Self-hypnosis for Change

Many different techniques can be used to induce a hypnotic state. What they all have in common, however, is that they make it possible for us to bypass the critical faculties of the conscious mind and go directly to the subconscious, where all changes will take place. For self-hypnosis, the ideal state for this to happen is when both body and mind are completely relaxed. Therefore, the gateway to hypnosis in this book is through relaxation. The benefits of relaxation itself cannot be praised enough, particularly with regard to its effect on anxiety. When you relax, physiological changes take place within the body – your heart rate slows down, your blood pressure normalizes, stress hormones are reduced and your body comes back into balance. You also experience a wonderful sense of wellbeing. This sort of physiological relaxation usually induces a light hypnosis. For self-hypnosis, the ideal state is when both body and mind are completely relaxed.

Deepening Hypnosis

Once you are physically relaxed, you can further deepen that state by focusing on achieving mental relaxation. When you are mentally relaxed, the mind becomes free of clutter and it feels as if absolutely nothing will disturb you. In this state, your perception is enhanced and your awareness is heightened. You may also find that any problems that are causing you anxiety are transcended and you become calm and balanced. If you're completely new to hypnosis, you'll find yourself entering a magical world that is unlike anything you may have experienced before.

There are hundreds of ways that you can deepen your hypnosis. The most common methods are breathing and counting, or imagining that you are on an elevator going down or you are walking down a flight of steps.

Post-hypnotic Suggestions

This is an extremely important part of self-hypnosis. A post-hypnotic suggestion is what you tell yourself, during hypnosis, in order to elicit the response you desire for the future. In essence, you are telling yourself how you should react after coming out of hypnosis. The suggestion is absorbed by the subconscious mind during hypnosis but acted on later. Suggestions could be words, images or symbols. They work like triggers so that any mention of the word, image or symbol in the appropriate context will bring on the desired response. It is important to be really clear and specific about what you wish to achieve and then create a strong sensory representation of how that will be. You also need to repeat and practise your post-hypnotic suggestion until it becomes an automatic response.

All post-hypnotic suggestions should be simple, realistic and in alignment with your belief system. They can be related to anything that you are working on or that you wish to change. In the case of anxiety, you need to give yourself hypnotic suggestions that will bring about calm, relaxed states of mind. For example:

When I awaken at the count of five I feel calm and at ease and I continue to do so over the coming weeks.

As you construct your suggestion in your mind, use all your senses and make it as compelling as possible by playing to your dominant representational system (see page 146).

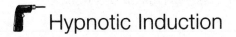 Hypnotic Induction

Now let's get practical. You can record the following techniques onto a tape or CD or listen to them on the pre-recorded CD. Although I have been encouraging you to use self-hypnosis, I do recognize that some people find listening to someone else's voice helpful when they first try hypnosis.

If you are recording your voice use 'you', as you will be relaying suggestions back to yourself. Use your chosen post-hypnotic suggestion once you are under hypnosis.

Step One – Your Breathing

The breath is a vital tool for achieving optimum relaxation and hence hypnosis. You can begin to control your mind and body by controlling your breathing. If you have a tendency to breathe in a shallow way you need to adjust your breathing to breathe more evenly and fully. Slow deep breathing triggers the relaxation response. When the body becomes relaxed physiological changes take place within it. As you breathe in, oxygen stimulates the brain and reaches all the cells in your body. As you breathe out carbon dioxide is expelled and tension is released.

As you do the following breathing exercise, be aware of the link between mind and body. A word of warning: do not breathe so deeply that you hyperventilate or your lungs hurt. It should be a relaxing process.

THE EXERCISE

Get into a comfortable position, either sitting on a chair or lying down. If you are sitting, ensure you sit with your back supported and feet firmly on the ground in an erect posture.

Take a deep breath down into your diaphragm, hold it for a few moments and then breathe out slowly, taking twice as long as you did to breathe in, and hold for a moment. Do it again – breathe in through the nose and out through the mouth. As you breathe in, use the whole of your lungs to fill every cell in your body with life-giving oxygen. Feel your ribs and abdomen lifting as you breathe in and falling as you breathe out, lifting as you breathe in and falling as you breathe out. As you breathe out, breathe away any tensions or feelings of anxieties that you might be holding. As you continue to breathe in this way, see the diaphragm like a bellows, contracting as you breathe in and relaxing as you breathe out. Expanding as you breathe in and deflating as you breathe out. Be aware of the sensations in your body as you focus your intention on the breath. Continue to breathe in this way and as you breathe, allow your lower chest, ribcage and abdomen to rise and fall evenly and naturally. You find that you are now relaxing deeper and deeper with every breath. Spend a few moments recreating this in your mind. See yourself relaxing more and more with every breath you take, see the lower chest and abdomen rising and falling with every breath you take.

Continue to breathe evenly, rhythmically and naturally and now, as you breathe, see the back of your body – see both the middle and upper back muscles expanding and falling just like the wings of a bird with every breath you take. Now see the breath spreading to all parts of your body, relaxing every cell. Pay attention to the sound of your breathing as you inhale and exhale. Hear the rhythm of the breath as you breathe in and out. Feel how relaxed you are now becoming as, with every out-breath, you go deeper into relaxation. Pay attention now to the sound of your breathing as you inhale and exhale. Give your breath a smooth rhythm as it rises and falls. Tell yourself with each deep, relaxing breath that you are feeling even more and more relaxed. Take your awareness to all the sensations in your body as you experience a warm flow of relaxation throughout the whole of your body.

Step Two – Muscle Relaxation

The next step is to relax all major muscle groups with different forms of progressive relaxation. The following technique is a fail-safe induction for almost everyone. Add the following exercise to the breathing one above. Ensure you avoid holding your breath in the following exercise. As you tighten your muscles, breathe in and as you let them go breathe out. As you breathe out you relax a little more by breathing away all the tension and tightness in your body.

THE EXERCISE

Begin by taking a number of breaths, inhaling through the nose and exhaling out through the mouth. As you do so, allow yourself to begin to relax and let go completely.

Begin by taking your attention down to your feet. Tighten the muscles in your feet. Feel your toes curling, hold this tension and then slowly let go for the count of 4. See your feet and toes relaxing completely: be aware of this – say to yourself 'my feet are relaxing now'. Follow the same procedure again and this time, study that tension as you tighten those muscles. Let them go and enjoy the comfortable feeling in your feet.

Now turn your attention to your calves. Tighten the muscles in your calves by trying to point your toes towards your face. Hold that feeling for a moment, now let go and relax those lower legs. Do it again. Tighten the calves, feel the tension and then let go and feel the relaxation flowing through those muscles right now. Say to yourself 'my calves are relaxed now'.

Turn your attention to your thighs. Raise your leg slightly and tighten those thigh muscles – the back, front, inner and outer.

Hold for a moment before lowering the legs and letting them go completely. Repeat this and notice how much more heavy and relaxed your legs are now feeling – your feet, calves and thighs. See the muscles in your calves and thighs completely relaxing – say to yourself 'my legs are relaxed now'.

Now pay attention to your buttocks and your lower back muscles. Squeeze them tight – see this happening in your mind and now let them go completely. Repeat this and as you let go of your buttocks and lower back see all tension leaving these muscles. Say 'my buttocks are relaxed now'. Feel any tension dissipating completely as your lower limbs now become heavier.

Now focus on your abdomen. Tense your stomach muscles by tightening them and pushing them outward. Feel that tension and now completely relax. Be aware of how completely relaxed your abdomen now feels. Repeat this, then say 'my tummy is relaxed now' and allow yourself to relax even more as you let go completely.

Now direct your attention to your chest and back muscles. Tighten the muscles in your chest – feel them tightening, see them tightening and hold for a count of 2. Now just allow your chest muscles to completely relax. Repeat this and say to yourself 'my chest muscles are relaxed completely'. Pay attention to your upper back muscles by squeezing the shoulder blades. See those back muscles tightening and now completely let them go and let them relax – say to yourself 'my chest and back muscles are completely relaxing now'. Repeat this.

Now tighten the muscles in your upper arms, lower arms, elbows and wrists and make fists with your hands. Imagine your arms are like steel rods. Hold for a moment or two. Now let go, allowing your arms to fall into your lap or hang loosely by your side supported by the floor or chair. See this in your mind. Say to yourself 'my arms are completely relaxed now, my hands are completely relaxed now'.

Now hunch up your shoulders – shrug them up towards your ears and tighten the muscles in your neck. Feel the tension in those shoulders. Hold for a moment or two. Now let go completely and allow your shoulders to settle in a comfortable position. Say to yourself 'my shoulders are completely relaxed now'. Feel the difference now that your shoulders are completely relaxed.

Now tighten all the muscles in your head and face. Tighten your scalp muscles and make a face. Scrunch up your forehead, your mouth, your eyes and try to scrunch up your ears. Hold for a count of four and now relax and let go completely.

Now focus your attention on the breath, inhaling and exhaling. Feel the waves of relaxation flowing like a warm blanket from the top of your head to the very tips of your toes.

Step Three – Mental Relaxation and Deepener

Once you are completely relaxed physically, you need to relax mentally. Again, you can record this exercise yourself or, if you prefer, you can listen to it on the accompanying CD.

THE EXERCISE

Imagine you are walking on a path that leads to a place of great beauty, peace and tranquillity. This path leads you to a gate. Beyond the gate, at the bottom of a flight of steps, is a place of paradise that will give you complete peace of mind. See yourself on the path right now, walking towards this place. You look forward to reaching your destination.

See what you see around you: perhaps beautiful colours, plants and animals – it's entirely up to you. All that you see fills you with pleasure. Hear what you hear – the sounds of nature, peaceful sounds, gentle sounds that relax you even more. Feel what you feel as you travel this path – peace and tranquillity with yourself and the world around you.

You now find yourself at the end of the path, going through the gate into the place that will give you even greater peace of mind.

As you enter the gate you feel the need to stop a moment and admire your surroundings. SEE WHAT YOU SEE, HEAR WHAT YOU HEAR AND FEEL WHAT YOU FEEL. As you admire your surroundings, you find yourself looking up into the sky. There you see a big white cloud floating by. You now begin to watch this cloud more closely and as you do so you notice a very strange thing. The cloud begins to take on the shapes of numbers. The numbers start from about 200 and then seem to transform to 199, then 198. You now begin to count these numbers and as you count you find yourself relaxing even more. The more you count the more you relax. Now the cloud is beginning to move on and fade away in the distance. As the cloud fades away so do the numbers. They get smaller and

smaller and you keep watching until they fade away completely. And even if you try to bring them back you find that they
just don't want to come. So you now choose to deepen your
relaxation by continuing your journey to paradise.

I'd like you to imagine that you are at the top of a flight of 20
steps. You take each step at a time and with each step you take
you double your relaxation. See yourself taking each step at a
time and relaxing your mind completely: twenty – you feel
more deeply relaxed; nineteen – going deeper and deeper again;
eighteen – even more deeply relaxed; seventeen – your limbs are
becoming heavier and heavier; sixteen – you now double your
relaxation; fifteen – with every breath you go deeper and deeper; fourteen – body and mind relaxing even more; thirteen – all
thoughts seem to fade away; twelve – with every breath you
take you go deeper; eleven – letting go now; ten – feel that
heavy floating feeling in your body as you relax even more; nine
– you are becoming closer and closer to complete relaxation;
eight – letting go even more; seven – even closer to complete
relaxation; six – every step you take you feel more and more at
ease; five – closer still to complete peace and tranquillity; four
– mind and body are on the verge of complete relaxation, that's
right letting go even more now; three – almost complete relaxation in mind and body; two – letting go completely now; one
– complete relaxation in mind and body. There, at the bottom
step, you find yourself in the most amazing place that you could
possibly imagine – it could be a sandy beach, a paradise island,
it's entirely up to you. You spend some moments now enjoying
the sheer beauty of this place. See what you see, hear what you
hear, feel what you feel. You again look for a place to sit and
you feel at peace with yourself and at peace with the world
around you.

After you have completed the physical and mental relaxation you then need to do the change work, either giving yourself suggestions for working towards your goal or moving towards the state that you want to achieve i.e. balance, calm and so on. To achieve your outcome you can use affirmations, visualizations or one of the mental exercises that involves self-hypnosis. If you haven't as yet decided on your desired outcome or the precise wording or image you want to use you should find the next chapter helpful.

Post-hypnotic Suggestion for Self-hypnosis

Now that you have experienced the power of the breath and the subconscious mind in bringing about optimum states of relaxation, you can use this at any time in the future to enter the state of hypnosis quickly and easily. All you have to do is take a deep breath and say the words 'relax now'. The deep breath and the words 'relax now' will take you to your perfect idyllic spot where you sat admiring the scenery around you. You then see the white cloud transforming into numbers again. Count them from 200 and allow yourself to relax deeper and deeper in between each number. You then deepen your relaxation by breathing deeply and taking yourself down that flight of steps to that amazing place. You do this easily and effortlessly until you slip into the right level of relaxation for you. Remember, simply the deep breath and the words hypnosis now will take you there.

Taking yourself out of Hypnosis

People often imagine that it is difficult to come out of hypnosis, when in fact awakening is the easiest part. I have never heard of anyone ever getting stuck in self-hypnosis. If an individual has difficulty coming out of hypnosis then it is most likely as a result of enjoying it so much they don't want to stop.

In the same way that you talk yourself into hypnosis, you can also talk yourself out of it. You do this by simply suggesting to yourself that you should awaken. There are numerous ways to do this. If, for instance, you have deepened your hypnosis by climbing down a flight of stairs, you can reverse that process and climb back up them again, all the while suggesting that it's time for you to awaken. If you wish to tape a suggestion for coming out of hypnosis, try the following (though do bear in mind that by recording this a set amount of time after your deep relaxation, you will be dictating the amount of time you spend in hypnosis – and some days you'll need more time and others less).

In a moment you are going to awaken with your subconscious mind having fully absorbed your suggestions. When you climb those 20 steps and reach the beginning of the path where you started from, you can open your eyes and become wide awake, full of energy and fully in the present. Let's start counting now: 1, 2, 3 – you now begin to feel a vibrant energy flowing through your fingers and toes; 4, 5, 6 – stretch those fingers and toes right now; 7, 8, 9 – feeling more refreshed and alert; 10, 11, 12 – be aware now of the sounds around you; 13, 14, 15 – feeling even more vibrant and alert; 16, 17, 18 – both mind and body are fully in the present now; 19, 20 – now you are walking up the path, hearing all the sounds from outside and in the room around you, you're becoming more and more awake and in the present with every step you take. That's right, now open your eyes and become wide-awake.

More Tools for Change

By now you should be aware of just how crucial language is to your state of mind. Positive suggestions made to the subconscious will promote positive action, if they correspond with your belief systems. As I've said before, the subconscious mind is goal-orientated and provides the energy and power to work towards the suggestions that you give it, irrespective of whether they're good or bad.

Unfortunately, on the whole, we are not taught to deal with negative experiences in a way that is helpful to us. The result is that when something challenging or threatening happens we immediately develop negative language patterns that we carry with us throughout life. What you think today will have an effect on how you will be tomorrow.

Thankfully, you can change those language patterns if you choose to. Remember, you weren't born thinking negatively – you have learned to do so in the same way that you have learned any other skill. If you have learnt something that is creating anxiety, you can unlearn it.

EXERCISE – CHANGE YOUR PATTERN

Make a decision to become more aware of what you are saying to yourself and the language pattern that you currently use. When negative language patterns pop up ask yourself 'where did I learn to think in this way?' Where did those current language patterns come from? Explore any negative beliefs that may come with this negative thinking and do the beliefs exercise on page 125 to change any limiting beliefs. Make a decision to stop negative language patterns. Take a deep breath and replace the negative with a more resourceful positive message instead. The more you practise this the easier the process will become.

After awareness comes action. It's time now to make your language more positive through the use of affirmations and scripts.

Affirmations

Affirmations are statements that you use all the time to assert your thinking. An affirmation is something you affirm to be true. They are very much linked to the beliefs and assumptions that we hold about ourselves. Affirmations can be incredibly empowering or disempowering, depending on your thinking. What is the difference between a suggestion and an affirmation? Suggestions create an impression or stimulate the mind, while affirmations are confident assertions of the truth or the existence of something. The following affirmations are typical of those that create anxiety:

I'm so stupid

I'm just not good enough

I'll never get this right

I'm so stressed out

I'll never lose that excess weight

I'll never be on time

I'm not loveable

I'll never make any money

I hate shopping

EXERCISE – BE POSITIVE

Put a different frame on the above statements. Take every one of these negative affirmations and turn them into positive ones. Flip them over to have the opposite meaning, so 'I'm so stupid' becomes 'I'm an intelligent human being and I'm learning every day'. Work your way through the list.

Now do a list of the negative things that you say to yourself and turn them into positive affirmations.

The better you feel about yourself, the less anxious you will feel and the more calm and relaxed you'll be. The more that you affirm that you are stressed and anxious, the more you'll become stressed and anxious. The more you tell yourself you are a failure, the more you become one. The more you agree about what you think others are saying about you, the more you are likely to create that reality. So it makes sense to repeat positive, supportive affirmations to yourself. If we repeat things to ourselves for long enough it soon becomes our regular dialogue.

Although you can use affirmations in self-hypnosis you can also write them down and stick them somewhere where you will see them often – on a mirror, a fridge door or on your office desk. Repeat them quietly to yourself. The more you affirm positive states of mind, the more likely you are to get them.

Watch Your Language

When you are making up affirmations choose your words carefully. There are certain words that are not useful – these include avoid, try, can't, won't, don't, perhaps, pain. When you use these words you are likely to formulate negative suggestions. So instead of saying 'I won't feel anxious and tired any more' try 'I am relaxed and calm and I feel full of energy'. Instead of 'I will try and avoid binge eating' you would say 'I eat in a calm and relaxed way'. Ensure you place a positive affirmation in your post-hypnotic suggestion.

EXERCISE – MAKE THE NEGATIVE POSITIVE

Think about your area of anxiety and make up an 'anti-anxiety script' – a positive statement of how your life is changing and improving (use the guidelines for positive language above). Fill your script with affirmations that you can tell yourself and repeat over and over again. If you are having difficulty, think about the opposite of the statement that you are currently using now – the following examples may be of some help.

★ Social Anxiety
   They hate me
   I know that I am not good enough
   They are judging me
      becomes...
   I respect and accept myself and others
   I feel warmth and friendship towards myself and others
   I have empathy for others

★ Fear of Failure
   I can't do this
   I am not good at this
   What is the point in trying?
      becomes...
   I know I can do this
   I'm growing more and more confident in my abilities every
      day
   I believe that all things are possible for me when I put my
      mind to it

★ Fear of Rejection
   I'm worthless
   I'm not loveable
   I hate myself
      becomes ...
   I am worthy of love and I love myself
   Every day I am becoming more and more secure within
      myself
   I am unique in my own way

★ *Relationship Anxieties*
  I'm hopeless in a relationship
  I know they think badly of me
  He/she is going to dump me
       becomes ...
  I communicate well in all my relationships
  I listen to everyone else's point of view
  I enjoy my relationships

★ *Learning Anxieties*
  I'm thick
  I'm just not able to grasp this concept
  I'm too slow
       becomes ...
  I learn easily and effortlessly
  I'm intelligent in my own way
  I concentrate easily and effortlessly

★ *Anxiety about Confidence*
  I can't carry this off
  I can't appear in front of all these people
  I'm not good enough
       becomes...
  I'm calm, confident, relaxed and capable
  My confidence grows every day
  I am now even more aware of my talents and my
     capabilities

Scripts

Scripts are a great way of feeding suggestions to your subconscious mind. They are simply a written copy of positive suggestions for the subconscious to accept during self-hypnosis. The idea is to focus on your areas of anxiety and write your own scenario, focusing specifically on the changes that you want to take place.

Using positive suggestions during self-hypnosis will enable you to reduce your anxiety levels more easily than you can imagine. In the state of self-hypnosis, what the subconscious mind accepts and believes to be true for you, it will do. I would strongly urge you to use self-hypnosis in all the different areas of your life – in your work, relationships, study, leisure and your health. It isn't just a means of countering anxiety – it will help you to reach all your goals in your life. Simply ask the question 'What do I want to change within myself?', write your script then go for it. Remember, your chosen script should be full of positive affirmations.

The following sample scripts – which cover some of the common causes of anxiety – are a good example of the sort of thing that you are aiming for. If you find any of these scripts appropriate to you, then by all means use them.

Everyday Anxieties

The feeling of calm is becoming more and more normal for you as you go about your daily life in a calm, confident way. Now, if anything comes up that causes you to feel tension, you take a deep breath and as you exhale you experience a sense of inner calm. As every day goes by you are able to rationalize your life in a calm way. You recognize that you have the most incredible potential to make every day an enjoyable one, if you choose. With this realization you find that you develop a much more positive outlook on life. You are confident in your decision-making. You feel in control of your life. You have complete control over your thoughts and feelings and this gives you a great feeling of calm and satisfaction – you are more accepting of others and their limits. You realize that there is good in people and you now look for those special qualities in others. You feel greater empathy with others and you direct your life in a way that benefits you and the world around you. As every day passes you become more and more relaxed within yourself and about yourself. These new positive feelings unleash your own natural creativity.

Confidence

Your confidence is growing every day. You are now even more aware of your abilities and you find ways to work on them. This new-found inner confidence enables you to feel stronger and stronger every day. These feelings stay with you always. All your special qualities are growing in every way. You recognize your true worth and this in itself generates confidence. Life now becomes so much more enjoyable, so much more fulfilling, as you feel more confident within. You exude confidence. You feel so much more secure about yourself. You now find that you are creating the life that you want. As you do this, the quality of your life keeps on improving. You have the confidence to carry through all your ideas. See yourself the way you wish to be – confident, relaxed, at ease in any situation.

Work Anxiety

See yourself relaxed at your desk. You concentrate easily and effortlessly. You are relaxed and confident that you can do all that you have to do in a calm and capable way. Your organization skills are getting better and better and you marvel at how easily and effortlessly you get things done. You find that you are calm at any meetings. You speak eloquently and articulately and you are confident that you have prepared for those meetings.

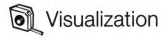 Visualization

By now you should be more aware that much of your thinking is visual and that you respond to the pictures that you make in your mind.

What your mind sees your body will do. This process provides us with yet another tool for transformation – the ability to consciously control our imagination. You can use your imagination to facilitate change in many areas of life. The conscious use of the imagination to achieve goals has been proven to be successful in many spheres, including sport, business, health and healing.

When you are consciously imagining, you are creating a clear image of something that you want to manifest. As you continue to focus on the imagined outcome you give it energy and create the neural pathways to make it happen.

Guidelines for Successful Visualization

★ Visualize what you really want. The clearer and more specific you can be about what you want to achieve, the more likely you are to get it.

★ Visualization is even more effective when the mind is in an optimum state such as hypnosis. You may also choose to visualize first thing in the morning or last thing at night, when the mind is in alpha or theta state.

★ When you visualize, use all your senses – words, images, feelings, smells, tastes and sounds. (Use the submodality exercises on pages 182–3).

★ Associate into your body when you visualize so you can experience the imagined scene as if you were really there.

★ Practise in your head to programme your neuromuscular pathways for success.

★ If you are visualizing a new behaviour, create a moving picture rather than a static one so that you are programming your neurology to do the actions as if they were real.

★ Make your visualization as detailed as possible to make your goal as compelling as possible.

Ensure that you are focusing on what you want and not on what you don't want. When we focus on situations that cause anxiety we often compound that anxiety because we can't stop thinking about the things that we're anxious about.

By now you will have created your own scripts in your given area of anxiety. At the end of your script of positive suggestions and affirmations, visualize how you wish to be. Create a visualization of new behaviours and positive states of mind.

EXERCISE – CREATE YOUR PERFECT SCENARIO

Imagine that you are in a cinema looking at the blank movie screen in front of you. Now allow an image of yourself, as you wish to be, to come up on that movie screen. See yourself calm, happy, relaxed, confident and handling whatever situation you have pictured yourself in. Make the picture perfect for you. Now step into the picture and fully associate into those feelings. Let them grow inside you. Just before the feelings peak, step out of the picture but imagine you are taking the feelings with you. As you now look at the image and feel these wonderful feelings, say your affirmation out loud. Use this affirmation as a trigger so that at any time you say the words in the future, your brain will associate the words with the picture you are making – and the positive feelings.

PRACTISE, PRACTISE, PRACTISE VISUALIZATION – IT TAKES JUST 21 DAYS TO CREATE A HABIT

Improving the Quality of your Experiences

We have already examined the way in which we use our senses and how vital they are in determining our emotional state. However, within the five senses are even finer distinctions that make up the quality of your experience. Whenever we make pictures, hear sounds or experience feelings we unconsciously break them down for storage and in the process 'code' them in a certain way. Crucially, the way you code an experience will have a profound effect on how you feel about it, adding intensity or momentum or making an experience more or less vivid. These small, specific aspects of our senses are called submodalities.

The Brain's Coding System

So what exactly are these finer distinctions that can so profoundly affect our thinking? When you have a sensory experience it usually has certain qualities to it, such as a location, size and shape. This is likely to be true for visual, auditory, kinaesthetic, odour and taste experiences (though the last two are not important in this context). Why, you may ask, are submodalities relevant? Because when you are aware of the submodalities you use you can start to change how you experience things. The following submodality distinctions are those that are most commonly experienced.

Visual Submodalities

Location – where is the picture located?
Number of images – how many images do you see?
Size – how big is the picture?
Shape – what shape is the picture?
Moving/still – is the image moving or still?
Colour/black and white – is the image colour or black and white?
Brightness – how bright is the picture?
Associated/dissociated – do you experience yourself inside the picture or as an observer to the picture? If observer, from what perspective do

you see this image?

Texture – does the image have a texture?

Distance – how far away is the image?

Contrast – what contrast of light and darkness does the image have?

Clarity – is the image in focus or out of focus?

Framing – does the image have a frame or a border around it?

Auditory Submodalities

Location – which direction does the sound come from?

Distance – how far away is the sound?

Words/noise/music – are you hearing words, noise or music?

Content – what are you hearing?

Loudness – how loud is it?

Tone/pitch – is it high pitched or low?

Clarity – is it clear or muffled?

Tempo – is it fast or slow?

Rhythm – does it have a beat or other kind of rhythm?

Mono or stereo – do you hear it one side or both sides?

Kinaesthetic Submodalities

Location – where do you feel it in your body?

Pressure – is there any pressure?

Temperature – is this sensation warm, cold or hot?

Texture – do these sensations feel smooth, rough etc.?

Moving/still – is there movement in the sensation?

Rhythm – is there any rhythm in the sensation?

Duration – is the sensation continuous or intermittent?

Speed – is it slow and steady or does the sensation move quickly?

I suggest that you copy out these submodalities so that you can begin to examine how you code experiences. By asking yourself these questions you can start to identify how you have interpreted situations. You can then set about changing those interpretations by altering the submodalities.

Self-hypnosis is a very useful state in which to change submodalities that are not helpful or useful to you. It's a bit like tuning the television or being a director of your own movie – when you direct your own brain, you can take charge of all the components that make up your experience.

EXERCISE – IDENTIFYING SUBMODALITIES

Think about a really pleasant experience. As you remember the experience, conjure up a picture of it in your mind. Look at the location in your mind, the shape, the size of the picture, listen for sounds, and tune into the tempo of the picture. Now focus on how this remembered experience makes you feel. Using the list of submodalities on pages 181–2, see if you can change that experience by changing the submodalities. (Remember its original picture so that you can change back again). As you change the submodalities be aware of which ones affect the memory the most and which ones affect it the least. If you wish, enhance the memory by changing the submodalities to make it even more pleasant.

Altering submodalities is not only useful for changing memories – it is also a good way of dealing with negative self-talk. 'You're such a dumbo' is a phrase I used to regularly repeat to myself. However, by changing the submodalities associated with this phrase I succeeded in altering its effect. When I hear that harsh voice, I change the voice and image of myself to that of Donald Duck or better still Betty Boop. This sounds incredibly comical and breaks the pattern. You can do the same in response to the negative dialogue that goes on in your head.

EXERCISE – ALTERING SUBMODALITIES

Think of an experience that makes you anxious. As you look at the picture, ask yourself 'what is the main submodality that is driving this experience for me?' If it feels stuck, make it a moving picture. If it is in your face, move it away into the distance. If a harsh internal voice sounds familiar, ask yourself whose it is. Recall somebody who has a warm loving voice instead. So now when you think about the critical things said, hear the warm loving voice instead. Notice how differently you are responding now. Be aware of how you feel as you make these changes. Be aware of how your state changes with the adjustments that you make. When the feeling is right, 'anchor' it in by thinking of a trigger word, symbol or action (for example, making a fist or even tweaking your ear). You can then use this at any time to trigger the brain to produce these new feelings.

EXERCISE – CHECK IT OUT IN REVERSE

Think of a memory that makes you feel anxious. As you focus on that image, see what you saw, hear what you heard and feel what you felt. When you get to the end of that experience run it backwards really quickly. Now think about the experience and notice the difference. When you reverse the order of an experience you can take the impact out of an anxious memory.

Association/Dissociation

Another excellent tool for self-hypnosis, and countering anxiety in general, is knowing when to associate with an experience and when to dissociate. When you associate with an experience you feel you are virtually a part of it – you see it and hear it through your own eyes and ears. When you dissociate, you assume the role of an observer. Whilst associating with an experience is great when it is a positive one, when the experience is negative it pays to have the ability to dissociate. This skill is crucial because it allows you to look at experiences you have had – to look at yourself as if you were an actor in a play – and make a dispassionate assessment of where you went wrong. By dissociating, you can look at things from a new angle, learn from your mistakes and decide how you can go about things differently in future.

EXERCISE – FILE THE JOKE

Think of an experience that really made you laugh. As you recall the experience, fully relive it by associating into the situation. See what you saw, hear what you heard, feel what you felt. Now imagine that you are floating out of your body and looking on this situation from an observer's point of view. How does it feel different? Float back into your body and allow your amusement to grow until you want to explode with mirth. Create a visual symbol – one that adds to the laughter – to represent this feeling and just recall it, and the associated feeling, whenever you need an instant lift.

Individuals use association and dissociation to varying degrees and in very different ways. Those who fully associate into all of life's experiences do so whether they are positive and negative. As a result, life can be a bit of a roller coaster ride – one minute it's fantastic but the next it's dreadful. If this applies to you, then you need to find ways of dissociating from situations that are a source of anxiety. In contrast, some people dissociate from both positive and negative experiences. However, whilst this means they avoid painful situations, it also guarantees the pleasurable ones are less enjoyable.

People who experience a lot of anxiety in their lives are often those who associate into the negative experiences and dissociate from the positive ones. When you think of it in this way, it sounds like a completely illogical thing to do. Yet so many people do it – they focus on the negative and seem to be unaware of all the positive aspects of their lives.

The happier, and possibly more successful, people in life dissociate from negative experiences and associate into the positive ones. They develop an ability to step back from experiences that are not useful and fully associate into the ones that are likely to result in a more positive outlook on life in general. You may be wondering if it is really such a good idea to dissociate from negative experiences. The answer is, in the short term, yes – if you use dissociation to learn from those experiences and find something positive in them. All you are doing is putting some mental and emotional distance between yourself and the experience in order to manage it better.

Getting the Balance Right
Clearly both association and dissociation can be harmful to your wellbeing if you use them inappropriately. When you are associated with an anxious state it can be difficult to get out of. In addition, in such circumstances, it's easy you find yourself setting up triggers and associations for the future. Hence any similar situation will evoke anxiety and the spiral will start all over again (for more on this see Anchoring, page 187).

We can't, however, spend all our lives avoiding painful feelings. If you permanently dissociate from particular feelings in this way you're not really dealing with them. If unpleasant feelings are causing havoc in your life it is important, at some point, to stay with those feelings if only to work out what they are about and how you can begin to deal with them.

In general, associating is good for learning and practising skills and enjoying pleasant experiences – past, present and future. Dissociation is a useful tool for stepping back from unpleasant situations and using the distance this provides to sort things out in your mind. In the time-line exercise on page 79 dissociation is used to avoid associating into any strong emotional events from the past.

RECOGNIZE WHEN YOU ARE ASSOCIATING AND DISSOCIATING

Recognizing the difference between when you are associating and dissociating allows you greater choice in managing your emotional state. Make a commitment to practise these two states and you will become even more aware of the difference.

EXERCISE – LISTEN TO YOUR OWN ADVICE

How are you feeling right now? Take a few deep breaths, step outside your body and take a good look at your physiology. How is your face? Is your forehead smooth and relaxed or is it furrowed and anxious? Is your jaw tense and anxious? How is your posture? If you are looking anxious, imagine that you are talking to that anxious person. Ask them what are they anxious about. Allow a wiser part of yourself to pass on some words of wisdom. Notice how the picture begins to change and transform into a much calmer you. Continue to offer those words of wisdom until all the muscles in the body seem to relax. Notice how your breathing has slowed down completely. Step inside your shoes again and associate into your relaxed calm body.

You can use these techniques in self-hypnosis and in your daily life to explore experiences and instigate positive changes. They can also be useful for mapping your future. In hypnosis, as your body relaxes, so does your mind, enhancing perception and awareness. In this state you can use both association and dissociation to solve problems. This gives you the foundations to make and create change where it is needed.

You will probably find yourself going into a light trance state as you work through many of these exercises. If, whilst exploring your experience, you encounter upsetting memories it can be useful to dissociate from them while allowing yourself to observe them (as in the timeline exercise on page 79). You can then change the submodalities to take the emotional intensity out of a memory – for example, if your memory is in glaring colour put a smoke screen in front to mute the colour or make it black and white.

From this position you can see what resources were needed back then and you can use these in the present, if necessary. You can also plan your goals for the future and associate into the future that you see for yourself.

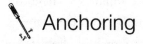 ## Anchoring

The final mental tool we will be using to counteract anxiety is a process called anchoring. An expansion of Pavlov's concept of associative conditioning, anchoring was developed in the late 1970s by Richard Bandler and John Grinder, the pioneers of NLP. As a result of their studies they came to the conclusion that it isn't just external sensory cues that trigger a particular response, an internal stimulus, such as a memory, can do this too. These cues, or stimuli, whether internal or external, are 'anchors' – they elicit a specific response or state of being.

Imagine for a moment that you're listening to the radio and a song comes on that you associate with a particular emotional event. As you hear the song you are transported back to that event and all the feelings that go with it. For you, that song will automatically produce that particular response because the two are intimately connected in your unconscious.

Everyday Anchors

In many ways life is just one big anchor. We create new anchors and we respond to old ones all the time. Anchors are easily established over a lifetime and we are often completely unaware of them. Your everyday anchors can be numerous: the smell of fresh coffee, a favourite perfume, a certain tone of voice, a particular word, an advertising jingle.

You will find anchors in every area of your life. In your immediate environment you will have set up anchors in the home (hopefully pleasurable ones) – think about your favourite chair, your bathroom, your garden. What about office anchors? Your office suit means it's time to focus on work; jeans means it is time to relax and play.

YOUR EVERYDAY ANCHORS CREATE YOU

Anchors work like light switches – the sensory stimulus switches on the specific neurological response. Anchors can be both positive and negative and they can often create extreme states such as phobias. An intense trauma can set up an anchor for life. This is because an association is made immediately because of the high emotion that comes with the event – and the more intense the experience the more powerful the anchor. Most anchors become established through repetition.

EXERCISE – WHICH ANCHORS ARE CAUSING YOU ANXIETY?

Think about the anchors in your life that create anxiety for you. Make a list of visual, auditory, kinaesthetic, olfactory and gustatory anchors that make you anxious. Here are some from my list:

★ *Wasps – these instantly make me panic*

★ *Loud music – this immediately triggers irritation*

★ *Deep water – not being able to feel my feet on the bottom automatically makes me anxious*

Obviously a degree of anxiety is perfectly normal and is difficult to avoid, as we respond to our anchors without thinking. However, that does not mean we cannot intervene in the process. Now that you are more aware of anchors, you can begin to recognize the triggers and make a decision to change them. You don't have to respond to sensory stimulus in the way that you do. You can create new anchors as a tool for self-empowerment and self-improvement. The following techniques can be used in or out of self-hypnosis (particularly when giving yourself a post-hypnotic cue for the future). When you start building more resourceful anchors you are imprinting good feelings and training your brain to respond differently.

Guidelines for Anchoring

★ Think about the state that you want.

★ Think of an experience in which you can see, hear and feel it.

★ An anchor should only be applied when you are fully associated in an intense state – i.e. when you are really 'in' the experience you are thinking about, seeing, hearing and feeling it.

★ You can create anchors using different representational systems, for example voice, tone, words, pictures or a physical act such as pinching fingers, making a fist or tweaking an ear.

★ Anchors need to be used for full effectiveness. If you do not use them they will fade. So repeat your anchors to make them even more powerful and effective.

★ Try to make your anchor unique – it should be different to what you do in your everyday environment.

★ Your anchor should fit with the context in which it is needed. Punching the air may be useful at the end of a game or privately, when you have succeeded at something, but not at the end of a presentation or in the middle of a lunch or dinner date.

★ Timing is everything – use your anchor as soon as you begin to think about the state you wish to anchor in, hold the anchor and when you see the state reach its peak let go – this could take anything between 5 and 15 seconds.

★ The more intense the emotion the more resourceful the state.

★ Always test the anchor that you set and check that it has worked. If it feels weak, go through the process again until you feel a difference (you may have to choose a more powerful experience).

EXERCISE – GETTING OUT OF A STUCK STATE

Think about an everyday anxious state that you would like to get out of. See what you are seeing in that state, hear what you are hearing and feel what you are feeling. Take yourself out of that state by looking around you or distracting yourself for a moment or two.

Now think about a positive state that would counteract the negative one. Recall the positive experience: relive it by stepping into your body and seeing what you saw, hearing what you heard and feeling what you felt. Fully associate into the experience. Allow the feelings to become more and more intense and bigger. As you begin to experience the intensity of these feelings, take your non-dominant hand and press the forefinger and thumb together; hold it for 5 to 15 seconds or until the state peaks. (Make sure you do not continue the gesture beyond the peak of the experience.)

Now take a break and distract yourself again.

Test your anchor by pressing forefinger and thumb together — the feelings should flood back. If you do not feel those feelings strongly enough, did you associate in the first place? Repeat the exercise and ensure that you associate fully.

Now think about the experience that makes you anxious and, as you experience those feelings again, press the forefinger and thumb together and notice how you can take yourself out of this anxious state.

EXERCISE – LOCKING IN NEW BEHAVIOUR

Imagine a challenging situation happening in the future. As the situation looms up be aware of how you feel and how you might have felt in the past. Ask yourself how would you rather behave and now imagine yourself behaving in that way. Make a really strong picture of how you wish to be by using your submodalities. Make the colours brighter, the picture clearer and put the picture in the location that seems right. Add some sound to the picture. Imagine that you are stepping into the picture and fully experience those new feelings and actions. Allow them to get bigger and bigger. Let the feeling get really intense and then step out of the picture and bring those strong feelings with you. Now turn and look at the picture and feel the compulsion to move towards it. Take your non-dominant hand and make a fist to lock those feelings and the associated picture in your body.

Now test it.

Think about the challenging experience. Now press the anchor and notice how your state and experience changes completely as you now focus on the new experience. What behaviours can you now put into place to ensure that calm, relaxed and in-control future you?

Anchors need to be repeated and reinforced. The more you practise these techniques the more you are conditioning your brain to work towards optimum states of wellbeing.

A Post-hypnotic Suggestion

You can also use anchoring post-hypnotically to anchor in resourceful states for the future. Do this by reminding yourself that you can, at any time you wish, trigger that state by using your anchor. This is an excellent way of automatically conditioning yourself to respond in a particular way to future situations.

Putting it all Together –

Your Anxiety Toolbox

By working through the previous chapters and doing the exercises they contain, you will have made a great start on tackling your anxiety. The purpose of this chapter is to pull together the exercises and therapies that are particularly relevant to each of the anxiety states discussed in chapter two and provide a summarized strategy for changing those states. The tools you need are at your fingertips – all you need to do is take a deep breath and make the decision to focus on what you want to achieve. These tools will help you to achieve that end. The scripts in this section are simply sample scripts to start you off. You now have the tools to begin to write your own.

 ## Anxiety/Depression

EXERCISE ONE – SETTING A NEW OUTCOME

Depression is often a vicious circle, with negative, self-defeating or sabotaging thoughts churning over and over again in your head. However, even in the depths of depression you can make a choice to move away from it. Even if you think you don't know specifically what you want, imagine that you do and go with whatever comes up. Sometimes it may just simply be to feel 'sunshine' again or to have peace of mind. These are as good places as any to start from, as you will begin to focus on the behaviours that you will need to do to achieve those states of mind. Do the Choose Your Outcome exercise on page 155.

EXERCISE TWO – TFT FOR
DEPRESSION/ANXIETY

If you are suffering from a combination of anxiety and depression, do Algorithm One (see page 116 or the CD). If you feel that depression is more of a problem do Algorithm Two (see page 117 or the CD).

EXERCISE THREE – CONFIDENCE
AND ESTEEM BUILDING

Often depression and anxiety are caused by a lack of confidence, poor self-esteem and limiting beliefs. TFT will have taken out the perturbation related to the cause of this. However, it will be useful for you now to explore a new way of thinking. Then you need to find new reference experiences to back up your new way of thinking. I would strongly suggest you work at a number of the other beliefs exercises in this book. The following exercise is also for building confidence and self-esteem. You could do this exercise in self-hypnosis and also add it to a confidence-building script or the depression/anxiety script.

1 *Write down the many times that you have performed well at a task, you were praised or were more than good enough.*
2 *Now choose the ones that you were most proud of.*
3 *If you wish you can put yourself into self-hypnosis. Imagine that you are in a cinema about to watch those experiences. You are playing the starring role.*
4 *Run the movies of those experiences – each one fully. As you watch these movies, one after another, adjust all the qualities in full colour. Further enhance them – make them brighter, larger, louder and more intense.*

5 *When you get to the end of these movies run them over again and make them even more perfect for you. Run the movie three or four times in total.*

6 *Come out of hypnosis.*

Now ask yourself what the special quality was that enabled you to succeed. What were the qualities that seemed to stand out in all of them? Use that quality as an affirmation – write it down in a bold colour and stick in as many places as possible, for example in your wallet, on the fridge, on your computer…

Think about how you want to be in the future. Make a picture and then bring these qualities to this picture. Step into the picture and fully associate into it – see what you are seeing, hear what you are hearing, feel what you are feeling. Allow these feelings to get bigger and bigger then step out of the picture but take the feelings with you. Turn and face the picture and make sure that it has all the qualities of your successful experiences. Anchor the picture and feelings so that in the future you can remind yourself that you have these qualities simply by using the anchor.

Practise using your anchor and visualize that future as often as possible.

EXERCISE FOUR – GAINING NEW LEARNINGS

1 *Think of a negative experience, related to anxiety or depression, that you want to change.*

2 *Remember that negative experience/behaviour.*

3 *Imagine a movie screen and run the movie of that experience. See yourself in that experience – see what you saw, hear what you heard, feel what you felt.*

4   How was that experience useful to you back then? What was it doing for you? If you don't know, then imagine you do.

5   As you look at this experience as an observer, what can you learn from it that will enable you to let go of any negative feelings, accept the intention of the behaviour and make a positive change for the future?

6   Think now about that experience. How do you feel about it now?

7   Apply what you have learned to another similar experience where that learning could have been beneficial. How is that experience now?

8   Use what you have learned to reshape future events in which it would be useful to act in this way. Notice the difference.

EXERCISE FIVE – AUTO SUGGESTION FOR DEPRESSION AND ANXIETY

This exercise is best recorded onto tape or CD.

Put yourself into self-hypnosis or deep relaxation.

As you rest, you become aware that moment-by-moment you are recovering your sense of proportion easily and effortlessly. Every day you have a greater sense of wellbeing and you now feel more positive within yourself and about yourself. As you continue to relax more and more with every day that passes, you begin to see and hear things in a different way. You develop a new perspective in many areas of your life. You now focus on the positive side of things in all areas of life and you now begin to feel more and more confident and positive about yourself. You find that with every day that goes by, your energy levels increase and you feel better and better. Your enthusiasm for life returns easily and effortlessly. Every day you feel a greater sense of vitality flowing through your body and mind.

Now, with the power of your imagination, see yourself as you wish to be – calm and relaxed. As you look at this picture, make it as compelling as you can by changing the qualities – make the picture brighter, bigger, make the sound perfect for you. Add some feeling to the picture – a sense of happiness and confidence and of being at peace with yourself. As you now see yourself as you wish to be, give your subconscious mind permission to continuously work towards this goal by giving this picture a big tick.

General Anxiety

The most prominent characteristic of GAD is the high level of worry that sufferers experience – they worry about the past, about the future and about real or imaginary problems. Whilst it's certainly normal for people to worry – and indeed it can motivate us to sort out problems – it is less helpful when worry becomes negative, as this has an effect on anxiety levels. When we become overly worried and anxious it is difficult to have a balanced perspective on life and, as a result, our view of situations and problems often becomes distorted and inaccurate.

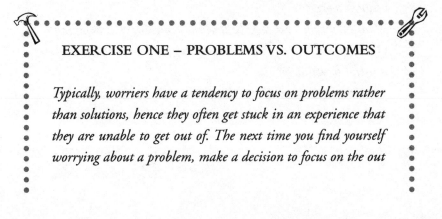

EXERCISE ONE – PROBLEMS VS. OUTCOMES

Typically, worriers have a tendency to focus on problems rather than solutions, hence they often get stuck in an experience that they are unable to get out of. The next time you find yourself worrying about a problem, make a decision to focus on the out come you want to achieve. This makes problems seem more like challenges. Do the Choose Your Outcome exercise on page 155.

EXERCISE TWO – CHALLENGING
YOUR BELIEFS ABOUT WORRY

It is very common to resist managing worry because of the belief that it helps to solve problems and protects us from danger. Yes, worry is normal to a certain degree but it becomes detrimental when it brings about ongoing anxiety and interferes with your life.

On a scale of one to 10, where one means of little use and ten is very useful, how much do you believe that worry is useful to you? Make a note of your answer.

Now explore your experience:
Ask yourself what worry does for you.
What do you value about worry? What do you not value?
How has worry affected your anxiety levels?
As you think about your experience would you say that worry has been helpful or harmful to you in your life?
What would it be like to believe that you could achieve greater balance and manage your life in ways other than through worry?
What might the next steps be towards achieving that balance?
On a scale of one to 10 how much do you believe that worry is useful to you now?
The next step is to recognize that facing your worries is the only way forward to emotional growth and reduced anxiety levels.

EXERCISE THREE – FACING YOUR WORRIES

1 *Sit in a comfortable position, one in which you can completely relax, and take a number of deep breaths. Now imagine a line of time floating into the future. Give it a colour. Now imagine yourself floating out of your body and travelling forward in time to when you are very old. Look back over your life at how much you have worried. Would you say that you have wasted too much time worrying? How has worrying affected your health, your relationships and your life? As you continue looking back, give yourself some feedback. When you have finished, float back to the present to receive that feedback.*

2 *Now, with this feedback, what do you think about your worrying. If you come to the conclusion that you have wasted a lot of time worrying, how can you begin to let go of worrying in the future?*

EXERCISE FOUR – THOUGHT FIELD THERAPY (TFT)

TFT is a very powerful technique for countering general anxiety. From your list of worries, pick the areas that you are most anxious about and do Algorithm One, which can be found on page 116 or on the CD.

EXERCISE FIVE – CONTROLLING WORRY

One of the greatest difficulties with managing GAD is that worrying can seem to take over your life completely. However, you can learn to catch it in the act.

Step One

Begin by keeping a record of your worrying thoughts. Do this for a week.

Note the date, situation and trigger, and describe the worry, the intensity of emotions, your response to the worry and, lastly, the outcome of your worry.

Look for any regular patterns that seem to be occurring. Make a decision to be more aware of your worry triggers and how you respond to them. Know that you do have a choice and can respond differently if you choose to.

Step Two

Choose one of your worrying thought patterns and imagine a movie screen in which you replay the situation that triggered it. Replay it in slow motion so that you can analyse that experience. See what you saw, hear what you heard and feel what you felt. What would you be seeing, hearing and feeling if you were to respond in a new way? Pick a few responses. What would you rather be doing instead? Now put these responses up on the movie screen and see what you see, hear what you hear and feel what you feel. Now choose the response that feels best. Take yourself through the situation again and intervene with the new response instead. Fully associate with this experience. Anchor it by either making a fist or using a word or symbol. Practise this new response, both in mind and body, every day by using your anchor as many times a day as possible and thinking about your new response.

EXERCISE SIX – SCRIPT FOR GENERAL ANXIETY

You will need to record the script for this exercise onto tape or CD (it's a little long to memorize).

Put yourself into self-hypnosis.

Now do a visualization. Imagine that you are going through a ritual of putting all your worries in a wooden box. When you have a sense that all your worries are in the box, imagine an incinerator with powerful flames. Pop that box in the incinerator and see the flames consuming the box. Watch them disappear from your life forever. Say the following affirmation:
I let go of worry in my life now and in the future.

Now listen to the following script:
Your subconscious mind is working powerfully on your behalf to ensure that you are relaxed and calm. With this new calmness and relaxed attitude you find that you handle situations so well. You manage your life in a new way. You recognize that worry is no longer a part of your life and you now find more useful ways to manage your everyday experiences. Your attitude is so much calmer towards others. You realize you are completely in control. You handle situations easily and effortlessly. You find that you are so much more accepting of your life and you feel so much better as you handle life in a calm, positive way. Your sense of humour returns as you become more attentive to other people. You recognize the opportunity in being so much more positive about yourself. You look forward to living your life in a very different way. With each day that passes you are happier than you have ever been before, knowing that you can look forward to the future with a calm relaxed mind. See yourself as you wish to be – relaxed, calm, at ease and happy with yourself. Take a deep breath and say the word 'calm' as you exhale. Whenever you need to be calm and relaxed in the future you simply say these words and this picture will come to your mind.

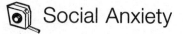 Social Anxiety

EXERCISE ONE – SETTING THE SCENE

So how do you overcome anxiety reactions in public or social situations? You begin by becoming very clear about what you want to achieve. The more specific you can be about what you want, the more likely you are to get it. So go through the Choose Your Outcome exercise on page ?? and define exactly what it is that you want.

For example:
I want to look my boss in the eye
I want to feel comfortable speaking in public
I want to give an excellent presentation

EXERCISE TWO – TFT FOR SOCIAL ANXIETY

The appropriate TFT treatment for social anxiety is Algorithm Three (see page 118 or the CD).

For most, using TFT will eliminate the perturbations in the thought field. This is usually enough to help you be more open to changing your beliefs about a given area of anxiety. The following exercise explores how you can challenge limiting beliefs and replace them with positive ones.

EXERCISE THREE – BELIEF CHANGE

Step One

Think of a belief that has held you back, for example 'I can never give a good presentation'. Now find at least three recent experiences that have proved this belief to be untrue – in other words, doubt its validity. For example, you might have told a really great story to your friends at dinner the other night, or you once gave a great presentation at work or a good perform- ance in the school play.

Step Two

Be open to believe something else. What would you rather begin to believe instead? Imagine that you are taking advice from a person you really like and admire. Imagine yourself by floating up out of your body and into theirs, surrounding yourself with their energy. Let them speak through you now.

Using their advice, think of a more useful belief that will replace the limiting one and open up new possibilities – i.e. 'I believe that as I work on my presentations I will get better and better'.

Step Three

Now think of an image or symbol to represent the old limiting belief. Imagine an old storage room – dark, dank and cob- webbed. Put that old belief in that room and leave it. Create an image or symbol to represent the new helpful belief and imagine that you have placed it somewhere in your home where you will see it all the time. Decide that every time you look at it you will be even more empowered by your new belief.

EXERCISE FOUR – BIOLOGY OF EXCELLENCE

This exercise is particularly good preparation for facing challenging social situations. You can act out this exercise or do it in your imagination.

1   *Choose a situation in which you wish to perform well socially.*

2   *Write down a list of resources that you need to be able to do this – i.e. confidence, strength, assertiveness, humour.*

3   *Think of an anchor that you can use – i.e. squeezing the fingers together, making a fist, tweaking your ear. Make it a discreet one.*

4   *Choose five of the most important resources and recall five experiences in your life when you had them.*

5   *In your imagination, see a shape – any shape you like (it could be a square, rectangle, triangle or circle of any size or colour). See that shape on the floor.*

6   *Think about the resource that would be most important to you. As you think about this resource recall the experience when you possessed it. Now step into the shape and relive that experience. See what you saw, hear what you heard, feel what you felt. Allow yourself to FULLY associate into the event. Allow the experience to increase in intensity. When you strongly feel the experience, anchor it. Leave the resource in the shape and step out of it now.*

7   *Repeat step 6 with all the other resources, using the same anchor.*

8   *When you have anchored all the resources in the shape step back into it and re-access all the resources by using your anchor. Feel that cocktail of positive resources flowing through you. Step out of the shape.*

9   *Think about a future situation where these resources would be useful then step into the shape, use your anchor and be in that future situation.*

10 *Now imagine folding up the shape into a tiny size that you can put in your pocket or in your mouth or wherever. When you need those resources in the future all you need to do is to take out your imaginary shape and tap into it using your anchor. (If it feels like you need to add some more useful internal states then do so.)*

EXERCISE FIVE – MODELLING NEW BEHAVIOUR

In order to change limiting behaviour, you need to think about how you are going to behave instead. If you are having difficulty in learning a new behaviour modelling someone you like and admire who has that behaviour can be helpful.

You can put yourself into self-hypnosis for this exercise and then do the script afterwards, expanding and filling it with your own personal suggestions.

Imagine a movie screen with that person up there behaving in the way you would like to. See what they are doing that is so different. Now step into the picture and imagine that you are taking on their energy and that you are becoming them. Start to practise the new behaviour. What does it look like, sound like and feel like? Start to practise it for real. Now imagine you are behaving in this way instead of them. Keep running it over and over again in your head until it automatically begins to become you.

Shyness Script

I am becoming more and more confident every day. I look forward to social situations and I know that I communicate well with others. I am completely in control of the situation. My attention now becomes focused on others and away from myself. I develop great empathy with others.

Panic Disorder

As I pointed out in previous chapters, panic attacks can be minimized or even eliminated altogether. As most of them are born in childhood, people often opt to do regression work in a bid to get to the bottom of their problem (if you do you must see a qualified practitioner). However, TFT techniques can be so successful that they negate the need for this sort of approach. Another very effective technique is the thought scrambler exercise, which helps to alleviate panic in minutes. These are just a few of the tools you'll find in this section, so let's get started.

EXERCISE ONE – TAKING RESPONSIBILITY

The first step is to take full responsibility for your panic attack and panicky behaviours. On the whole we are a society that is not geared towards taking responsibility and often we look outside ourselves for the answers. It is certainly a possibility that external factors, such as poor nutrition or toxic substances, can have an effect. However, it may be useful for you to explore what else is happening in other areas of your life. After all, you were not born with a panic disorder, you developed it somewhere along the way. Explore your experience – do you, for example, become mentally and emotionally fatigued easily? Do you suffer from other types of anxiety or depression? Do you generally think positively or negatively about life?

After thinking about your experience, write down what you want to achieve. If it helps you to form your goal, do the Choose Your Outcome exercise on page 155. Typical goals for someone who has panic attacks might be:

I want to be able to manage my emotions more easily

I want to be free of panicking and more confident in myself

EXERCISE TWO – TFT FOR PANIC ATTACKS

The appropriate TFT treatment for panic attacks is Algorithm Three (see page 118 or the CD). Remember, you must tune into the anxiety that brings on the feeling of panic as you do the TFT treatment.

EXERCISE THREE – THE THOUGHT SCRAMBLER

This very simple technique is used in NLP. It can change an emotional state very easily and can therefore be used for any anxiety disorder, or strong emotions such as anger. You will need someone to help you do this exercise – so teach it to your friends, family or close workmates so that they can help you if necessary.

1 *First get your partner to assess your level of distress according to the SUD scale.*

2 *As you are experiencing distress, or thinking about it, your partner takes their finger 12 inches away from your face, points their finger at you and begins drawing a figure of eight quickly. You have to follow that figure of eight, focusing all your attention with your eyes. Your partner can make other shapes too, but they must do this quickly with their finger. You continue to follow their finger with your eyes.*

3 *After about a minute, your partner should ask you to assess what your level of distress is now and to think about what was distressing you. It's very likely that you'll have a considerably lower score, which means that the thought has been scrambled. If the level of distress has not dropped considerably then continue the finger technique.*

EXERCISE FOUR – INSTALLING A NEW BEHAVIOUR

Now you've gotten rid of that panicky feeling, you can install a new thought instead. The following technique helps train the brain to go in a new direction.

1 *Take your eyes down to the left, the area where you normally do your internalizing, and repeat a positive statement out loud – for example, 'I am calm, confident and relaxed'.*

2 *Now take your eyes from there up to the right. This is where we visually construct information. See yourself calm and relaxed. See what it looks like. Give yourself a strong visual image of how that might be – for example, I see a picture of me calm and relaxed and in fact I'm laughing.*

3 *Now take your eyes down and right and just notice how it feels. It should feel great, so say out loud 'it feels great'.*

4 *Now repeat the whole process again two more times, each time saying the statement with more feeling. Use the submodalities to make the picture bigger, stronger and brighter in whatever way is most compelling for you. Take your eyes down and feel it.*

5 *Make a commitment to practise this exercise until the new behaviour becomes habitual.*

EXERCISE FIVE – COUNTERACTING NEGATIVE STATES

The purpose of this exercise is to allow you to choose to respond in a more resourceful way in any given situation. By closely associating a negative and a positive state and making the positive one stronger, you make it easier to choose the more resourceful reaction. Each state is anchored by using a different location on the body – I recommend that you use opposites i.e. right knee and left knee or arms or different fingers.

Firstly think of a negative state that you want to counteract. Now think of a positive state or a number of positive states that you would rather feel instead. Recall a time when you experienced this state – see what you saw, hear what you heard, feel what you felt. Start adding other positive states and anchor all of them in the same location. Take a few deep breaths and distract yourself.

Now test the anchor.

Are you seeing, hearing and feeling what you want? If so, proceed. If not, go back to adding appropriate states. (Make sure that you fully associate into them.)

Now think about the negative experience. As you recall that experience see what you saw, hear what you heard, feel what you felt. Anchor this state just once in a completely different location. Take a few deep breaths and distract yourself.

Now test the anchor.

You should now have anchored in a negative state and a positive one in two different locations. The positive anchor should be a powerful state and the negative one weaker. Now use both your anchors simultaneously. Allow both states to peak – you will now have a sense of a change taking place. Take your hand off the negative anchor and keep your hand on the positive one for a few more seconds.

Now touch the negative anchor and be aware of how you feel. You will find that you will not respond to the anchor in the old un-resourceful way. The state should feel more neutral or positive.

If there are any remnants of the old state left, continue adding positive resource states and using your anchors until there is no negative state left.

EXERCISE SIX – CHANGING THE
NEGATIVE SELF-TALK

Negative thought processes play an enormous part in panic attacks so it is vital to take control of your thinking and change the words that you use from negative to positive. In this exercise, you choose positive language and visualize what those words mean (remember to use the guidelines for suggestion in chapter 7). The added benefit of this exercise is that it produces the relaxation response and this decreases the levels of blood lactate that, in excess, can make you feel very panicky.

Step One
Whenever something happens that causes you to feel panicky or tense and anxious, stop what you are doing, take a slow full breath (not too deep), inhaling through the nose and filling your lungs and diaphragm with air. Now exhale. Use this breath as an anchor to intervene and break this state. Now spend a few moments listening to what you are saying to yourself...

Automatic thoughts come as words, pictures and sensations. Be aware of how these thoughts are affecting you now.

Write down the thoughts you are having and how they affect you – for example, 'my heart is beating so fast I think I'm going to have a heart attack. The more I focus on my heart beating fast the faster it seems to beat.'

Step Two
Do you still want to have those thoughts? Are they useful or helpful to you? What would you rather think instead? Make a list of thoughts that you would rather have instead – for example, 'my heart may be beating fast but it will soon slow down and beat more normally'

Step Three
Now bring your other sensory skills into the equation. Say your new thought and now visualize it. Visualize your heart beating more slowly. Say to yourself 'my heart is beating at its natural rhythm now and I see it doing just that.'

Obsessive Compulsive Disorder

The main characteristics of OCD are the obsessions and the compulsions that occur in response to negative and persistent thought patterns. These contribute to a vicious circle of doubt and anxiety that results in behaviour that seems very difficult to challenge. However, the good news is that you can change this behaviour.

The first step is to focus on what you want to achieve. You then need to explore your beliefs and neutralize the obsession through TFT. At this point you can work towards creating a new strategy for situations that may have created anxiety and compulsive behaviour in the past. You then practise this new sequence of thought and behaviour, time and time again.

EXERCISE ONE – DECIDE WHAT YOU WANT TO ACHIEVE

The outcome you want will be personal to you, so the best way of deciding on this is to do the Choose Your Outcome exercise on page 155. A typical outcome might be something along the lines of:
'When I have turned the oven off I want to know and trust that I have done it so that I can get on with living my life. I would like to have achieved this by next week.'

EXERCISE TWO – BELIEFS EXERCISE

This exercise will help you to explore your existing beliefs and hence understand their deeper meaning so that you can challenge them and form a new perspective.

As you think about your obsession what is the belief or assumption that you hold to be true? Then ask yourself why that is a problem. For example:
I will always forget to turn the oven off
Why is that a problem?
I will simply never remember to turn it off
Why is that a problem?
Well, I might come home to a house full of gas
Why is that a problem?
It would be unsafe
Why is that a problem?
I don't like feeling unsafe
Why is that a problem?
I feel unsafe a lot
Why is that a problem?
I feel unsafe outside
And why is that a problem?
The world is an unsafe place

Be open to believe something else instead
How can you begin to challenge this belief and find positive ways of operating in the world to feel safe? Where does this belief come from?

Cast your mind back to its possible origins and, as the answers pop into your mind, explore the answers from an observer's point of view. What is there for you to learn from this that will enable you to begin to loosen the hold that your current belief has on you? If you were to advise that younger you, what would you say to yourself?

Designing A New Belief
What would you rather believe instead? What do you need to believe in order to achieve your outcome? What are the first steps towards deepening this new belief? For example, 'the world isn't always scary and I can learn to cope better'. Find experiences that back up this new belief.

EXERCISE THREE – TFT FOR OBSESSION

The appropriate TFT treatment for OCD is Algorithm One (see page 116 or the CD).

EXERCISE FOUR – STRATEGIES

We have strategies for everything – eating, drinking, making love; you run strategies in your relationships, you have a decision-making strategy, a motivation strategy. You also have a strategy for your compulsive behaviour.

An excellent way to describe strategies is to equate them to baking a cake or cooking to recipe. You need ingredients and each of the ingredients is added in a certain sequence to get the desired result. Therefore, in order to tackle your compulsive behaviour, you must somehow intervene in that strategy with something convincing enough to break it. One client of mine, whose obsession was turning the light switches in his house on or off, used what was for him a convincing symbol – he saw the switch as a pyramid. An upside down pyramid meant that the light was switched on and when the pyramid was the right way up it meant it was definitely switched off.

The purpose of this exercise is to discover what your current OCD strategy is and how you can successfully intervene to stop it. The exercise is best done with a friend (though you can do it by yourself). Get your friend to go through steps one to six with you. Your friend should be following the instructions below while you do what they ask.

1 Familiarize yourself with the information on eye accessing cues (see page 147) so that you can observe what your friend is seeing, hearing or feeling as they go over their strategy.

2 Ask them to act out what they do or to go through it step-by-step in their heads and describe it to you. Ask them to fully associate into what they do i.e. to relive exactly what happens when they do it. Ask them if what they are doing relates to what they see, hear or feel on the outside or is it something they make up or remember on the inside – i.e. do they see a picture or hear something in their mind?

3 Ask 'what is the first thing that happens, what happens next, what you are seeing, hearing or feeling?' Write down their answers.

4 As they go through their strategy, work out where they become stuck – i.e. at which point can they no longer exit from the strategy.

5 Give them feedback by backtracking over what they have told you. Make sure you focus on the process and not the content – for example 'so you did this and then you did this, then this and this'. If you like, act it out for them.

6 Find out if there is something they need to see, hear or feel in order to be convinced that they have completed the task. Ask how they know that they have completed the strategy. Again write down your findings.

At this point, the OCD sufferer takes over. Examine the notes your friend has made and begin to think about where you can intervene before your strategy starts to go wrong.

You may want to model yourself on someone else who has successfully taken themselves out of their compulsion loop. However, you need to design your own strategy by establishing a new sequence of events. Anchor these events spatially by moving from one step to the other.

Mentally rehearse the sequence, using all your senses. When you have completed the sequence in your head start the sequence again and this time make it bigger, brighter and add sound feeling etc. Now physically go through the sequence of events.

EXERCISE FIVE – PACING THE FUTURE

Go into self-hypnosis. Imagine a line of time that stretches out into the future. Float out into the future to a time when you will have successfully gotten over your obsessions and compulsive behaviour. Look back now on these old feelings; this old behaviour. Where is the anxiety now?

Now think about the new belief you have and strategy that you have learnt. See yourself performing this compelling sequence in your head with your new belief firmly in place. Make a powerful picture using all your senses. Put a frame around it. See yourself floating into the future with this picture and place it at that future time to remind your subconscious mind to work towards this goal.

Body Dysmorphic Disorder

If you suffer from BDD it is important to recognize that the perceptions you have of your self-image are a reflection of your own inner conflict. The view you hold about yourself and your body is heavily influenced by your experience to date – your likes, dislikes, beliefs and values. Your self-image develops into a framework out of which you create a picture of yourself as you understand and believe yourself to be. If this framework is distorted, you need to develop a more realistic assessment of yourself – you need to be more accepting of yourself whilst at the same time working towards being the best that you can be.

EXERCISE ONE – CHOOSE YOUR GOAL

Set your outcome – what do you want to achieve? Be realistic in your goal-setting; unrealistic expectations will only create anxious behaviour. Do the Choose Your Outcome exercise on page 155.

EXERCISE TWO – PERCEPTION IS PROJECTION

An excellent way to learn more about yourself is to monitor your thoughts about others. Often what we see in others we are really recognizing in ourselves. If you feel good about yourself you are likely to be less critical and judgemental of others. If you feel bad about yourself you are more likely to be critical and judgemental.

Over the next few days monitor your thoughts. Think about what you perceive in others and therefore in yourself. What generalizations are you making? What are you most critical about?

What judgements are you making? Where did you learn them? What does this exercise teach you about yourself?

If you were to change your thinking how could you begin to put a different perspective on your thoughts? Start to reframe your thinking. Perhaps you could begin by taking full responsibility for the way that you feel about yourself and by making the decision to move away from thinking that is not useful to you. You may choose to be more accepting of others and therefore of yourself.

EXERCISE THREE – GET A NEW PERSPECTIVE

Very often our views are heavily influenced by those around us. When it comes to the body, too many of us are swayed by society's view of what is perfect and what is not. Know that each and every individual is unique and although society sets the template there is nothing that says you have to follow it. Life is very much what it is. You cannot change society's view but you can change your own.

1 *Take a look in the mirror and think about the way that you feel about your body. Think about the beliefs that you currently hold.*
2 *Imagine a line of time that reaches out into the future. See yourself floating along into the future – to six months from now. Float into that you in the future and find yourself in front of another mirror. What do you see, hear and feel about yourself? What are others saying about you?*
3 *Float up above the timeline again to five years in the future and then down into the image of the future you. What do you see, hear and feel. What are others saying about you?*

4 *Now float up above the timeline to 10 years in the future, still retaining your current way of thinking. Float into the future you. What do you see, hear and feel about yourself. What are other people saying about you? Recognize the results you will get in the future if you continue to think in this limiting way about your body.*

5 *Take a break – stand up, sit down, turn around, it's entirely up to you.*

6 *What would you rather think or believe that would allow you to let go of your anxiety about your body image? Write down your answer.*

7 *Imagine now floating above your timeline 15 minutes after you have let go of the anxiety and limiting belief and having installed your new belief instead. Now, looking back, where is the anxiety now? What is your current thinking? With this new thinking take yourself into the future 6 months, a year, 5 years. How will your life be different now?*

EXERCISE FOUR – TFT TREATMENT FOR BODY DYSMORPHIC DISORDER

The appropriate treatment for this type of anxiety is Algorithm One (see page 116 or the CD).

EXERCISE FIVE – CHANGING YOUR LANGUAGE

You are the person you are today because you tell yourself every minute of every day precisely who you are. Over the next few days monitor the things that you say to yourself about your body image. Jot down what you hear.

How can you begin to change your language? Think about the comments you make to yourself most often. Change them to a more positive affirmation instead. Make a commitment to intervene on any negative dialogue in the future and use your positive affirmations instead. You may want to write down those affirmations and put them in obvious places so you see them all the time. Say your affirmations out loud and mean them. Keep on saying those affirmations until you really begin to believe them.

Use the following script for self-hypnosis (if it's a little long to memorize, record it).

Script
You have now experienced your subconscious mind helping you be the best that you can be. And you now recognize that the true path to feeling happy within yourself is through self-acceptance. Now become aware of your natural body shape; be aware of its natural contours. You recognize that we are all different shapes and sizes and each is beautiful and unique in its own way. You now accept the shape that you were born with and you become increasingly aware that you can be the best that you can be within that shape.

Phobias

If you have a phobia, the first thing you need to pinpoint is whether it is specific to one object or situation or if it is a more complex one. Those of you who have phobic responses or extreme anxieties in various situations are likely to have a more complex phobia and whilst the tools in this book can help, be aware that you may need more professional help to get to the bottom of them.

EXERCISE ONE – FACE YOUR PHOBIA

Stop avoiding the thing that you fear. You have survived so far and you can release this phobia with the techniques in this section. Focus on what you want to achieve. State the outcome you wish to achieve – for example, I want to be able to enjoy flying or I want to remain neutral to spiders. Work through the Choose Your Outcome exercise on page 155.

EXERCISE TWO – TFT TREATMENT FOR PHOBIAS

There are hundreds of different phobias. Here are just some of those that you can use TFT for: flying phobia, animal phobias, bird phobia, blushing phobia, monophobia (fear of being alone), driving phobia, water phobia, eating and food phobias, hospital phobias, illness phobias (fear of vomiting etc.), insect phobias, spider phobia, sexual phobias.

The appropriate treatment for phobias is Algorithm One (see page 116 or the CD). Remember, if TFT is to be successful, you must tune into the phobia that you wish to eliminate.

EXERCISE THREE – THE PHOBIA CURE

This is an alternative to TFT. It is a very quick and effective method of breaking the association between the object and the feelings it usually engenders. You can memorize the exercise, record it onto tape or CD or do it with a friend.

Firstly think about your phobia on a scale of one to 10. How much do you feel this phobia now? Take a few deep breaths or walk around the room to break your state. Put yourself into self-hypnosis or simply a relaxed frame of mind through doing the breathing and physiological relaxation (see pages 160–64)

1   *Imagine that you are sitting in the middle of a cinema. Up on the screen is a blank white screen.*

2   *Recall a situation that happened just before you had the experience that created the phobic reaction. Change the submodalities of this experience to make them black and white, and make it a still picture.*

3   *Now imagine that you are floating up out of your body towards the projection booth right at the very back of the cinema. As you find yourself in the projection booth, watch yourself still sitting in the cinema watching yourself on the screen.*

4   *Turn that picture on the screen into a black and white movie and run the movie of that phobic experience from the beginning to the end when all turned out well.*

5   *When you get to the end, when all was well, imagine that you are stopping the movie. Now imagine that you are jumping into the picture. Make the picture full colour and then very quickly (in no more than a second and a half) run the movie backwards. Do these steps a few times if you think it necessary. Make sure you end up where you started. Stand up now and walk around the room.*

6   *Think how you feel about that experience right now on a scale of one to 10 (10 being the worst). What is the difference? If the score is higher than 2 repeat the whole process, making sure you go through each step carefully.*

EXERCISE FOUR – FUTURE PACING

The objective of this exercise is to check if the previous techniques have worked. You do this by imagining a number of situations in the future and thinking about how you will feel and behave.

Take yourself to a future situation that, in the past, you may have had a strong negative emotional reaction to. Notice how it is different from your previous experiences in such situations. See what you see, hear what you hear and feel what you feel. Take a deep breath and take yourself out of this experience. Now take yourself to another situation and check again. See yourself as you would wish to be, hear what you would like to hear, feel what you would like to feel – calm, relaxed, perhaps even laughing at the thing that you feared. Imagine the situation as you wish it to be.

EXERCISE FIVE – SELF-HYPNOSIS
FOR TRAVEL PHOBIA

Travel phobia is particularly common, hence this specific exercise. It should be performed after TFT or the Fast Phobia Cure. You will need to record it onto tape or CD.

Put yourself into self-hypnosis and deepen your relaxation to the optimum level for you. Now, with the changes that have taken place, you feel calmer and calmer every day and you now look forward to travelling as often as you can. You look forward to all the exciting things there are to learn and see in the world as you now enjoy your travelling experience. And because of this you find that you are gaining so much more confidence within yourself and in your ability to travel easily and effortlessly. You find that you hear yourself saying I enjoy travel; I look forward to travelling. You ensure that you are well prepared for your journey and you feel safe because you have prepared so well. Imagine yourself at the airport/seaport/station waiting to travel; see yourself getting on board the plane/boat/train and telling yourself this is easy. You feel relaxed and calm. See yourself enjoying the journey in a calm and relaxed way. As you create this picture of yourself travelling, make it as compelling as possible. Make it as bright as you can, as strong as you can. Put the picture in a number of different locations in your mind to find the most compelling one. Now let the picture get bigger and bigger until you find yourself in the picture, fully associating into those feelings. Let the feeling become intense and imagine stepping out of the picture but taking these feelings with you.

Lock in these feelings by setting a kinaesthetic anchor such as tweaking your earlobe. Now, every time you tweak you earlobe, you tune into these fab feelings and this positive picture you have in your mind.

REMEMBER, AVOIDING THE THING THAT YOU FEAR ONLY PREVENTS YOU FROM UNLEARNING THAT FEAR

Health Anxiety (Hypochondria)

A great deal of light has recently been shed on this often-neglected anxiety. It is now understood that every thought we have has a physiological response in the body, hence sufferers of health anxiety are often expressing what is happening within them emotionally through physical symptoms. So although you may not have an illness, you are not necessarily imagining your symptoms.

Like all anxieties, health anxiety can be eliminated or minimized. Once you have been given a clean bill of health – in other words, there is no physical explanation for your problem – you need to recognize that your illness has non-physical components to it and you therefore need a greater understanding of how your mind works and the psychology of ill health. The first step is to explore any underlying beliefs that you have about your health.

EXERCISE ONE – EXPLORE YOUR BELIEFS

1 *Explore your experience with your health. What is your track record so far? Do you visit the doctor every time you have a physical sensation?*

2 *What else could be happening in your life at the time of your symptoms? Explore the events in your life leading up to this illness, what is happening in your life now and what do you foresee happening in the future?*

3 *Explore your current lifestyle habits. Are you drinking, smoking or taking drugs; do you have a poor diet? Could this be affecting your condition?*

4 *After you have been to the doctor and have been reassured, what happens to your symptoms? Do you become symptom free?*

5 *Based on the evidence that you have been given by the doctor, and through exploring your experience, what is your understanding of your condition now?*

6 *If you continue to believe that there is something wrong with you when all evidence suggests that there is not, what do you*

think your life is going to be like in the future? Take yourself forward 5 years, 10 years, 20 years.

7 *The next time you get a symptom, record its characteristics for a week: note the intensity, the location, whether it is there all the time or only occasionally. Notice if the symptoms lessen through the week.*

8 *Suppressing emotions – not the emotion itself – can damage your health. Next time you get a symptom of poor health ask yourself what this symptom is really telling you. What is it that you really fear?*

EXERCISE TWO – SETTING AN OUTCOME

If you accept your health anxiety and you believe that it is out of your control then you are likely to continue to have aches and pains and possibly create the very thing you fear. In contrast, if you believe that your health is under your control, this opens up all kinds of possibilities. Remember, you get what you focus on. Can you create your own desired outcome for perfect health for you? Set an outcome now. For example:
– I want a strong healthy heart
– I want to manage my stress levels better
– I want to believe that I can have optimum health
Do the Choose Your Outcome exercise on page 155. Have a clear picture of your outcome.

EXERCISE THREE – LOOSENING YOUR BELIEFS

If a doctor has reassured you that there is nothing physically wrong with you, then your beliefs and assumptions about your health are creating your current anxiety and quite possibly your current condition. In order to make a difference you need to revise your current beliefs, replacing them with ones that are empowering.

1   *Think about a belief that you know to be absolutely true for you – for example, 'I love my son'.*

2   *As you think about this belief, make a picture that represents it. Allow pictures, sounds and feelings to come flooding into your mind.*

3   *As you see this picture in your mind, elicit the submodalities of it – those finer qualities such as colour, size, sound etc.*

4   *Let your mind go blank.*

5   *Now think about something that you doubt is true. It can be something that is pretty obvious like 'there are aliens on Mars'.*

6   *Do the same as steps 2 and 3.*

7   *Let your mind go blank.*

8   *Now compare the two pictures and notice the differences. What seem to be the main submodality differences between them?*

9   *Think of a disempowering belief you have about your health that you want to change.*

10   *Create a picture that represents this disempowering belief and elicit the submodalities.*

11   *Take the submodalities from the earlier statement that you doubted and apply them to the negative belief you have about your health. How do you feel now about this disempowering belief? You should begin to doubt it.*

12   *Think of a belief that you would rather have instead – one that is exactly the opposite of the disempowered belief. Apply the submodality differences from the belief in step 1.*

Now what are your beliefs about your health?

EXERCISE FOUR – TFT FOR HEALTH ANXIETY

The appropriate treatment for this type of anxiety is Algorithm Three (see page 118 or the CD).

EXERCISE FIVE – DO YOU INVITE ILL HEALTH?

As you now know, we can influence our body simply with the language we use. Use a certain phrase often enough and you might well get what you ask for. Consider the following phrases:
He gets my back up
He's a pain in the backside
What a pain in the neck
That drives me nuts

Make a note of the terms you use. Think about your own mind–body experience. Have any of these or your own terms become true for you?

Clearly the language you use has a powerful effect on the physical body, as the emotion it brings affects many of the body's systems. It therefore makes good sense to use positive suggestions for good health and vitality. For example:

I have more energy and vitality every day
I enjoy exercise and I only eat foods that are good for my body
I believe every day I am getting better and better
I take care of my body and mind

Add your own affirmations to this list.

Post-Traumatic Stress Disorder

PTSD is somewhat different from other anxiety disorders. However, just as I encourage those who suffer from phobias, panic attacks, OCD and so on to confront their feelings, I urge PTSD sufferers to do the same. The more you try and push unpleasant memories away, the more they will come back to haunt you. And there are methods that help enormously with trauma. TFT can give outstanding results and at the very least be helpful. Techniques that dissociate and desensitize memories help enormously too. A TFT algorithm for trauma is included in the exercises but I strongly recommend Dr Callahan's books for more algorithms related to trauma and the emotions that come with it, for example guilt and anger.

Please note: these exercises do not take the place of professional help and if you are suffering from PTSD badly, your first stop must always be with the medical profession.

EXERCISE ONE – SET YOUR GOAL

Think about what you wish to achieve. Remember, the subconscious mind is like a heat-seeking missile and will respond to your suggestions – so the clearer and more focused you can be the better. Your goal does not need to be complex – 'I want to feel more emotionally balanced' or 'I want to be calm in the face of all my memories' are perfectly acceptable targets. Do the Choose Your Outcome exercise on page 155 to help you with this process.

EXERCISE TWO – TFT FOR TRAUMA

The appropriate treatment for trauma is Algorithm Three (see page 118 or the CD). Bear in mind that the brief amount of distress inherent in thinking about your area of trauma will be well worth it for the long-term benefits that you will achieve.

EXERCISE THREE – DISSOCIATING THROUGH POSTURE

PTSD sufferers often find themselves reliving traumatic experiences. TFT will have taken the sting out of PTSD, but learning how to dissociate will enable you to neutralize and reduce any negative feelings that may remain.

We adopt different postures for when we associate and dissociate, therefore adopting the appropriate posture can help with the process of dissociation.

Sit in a straight-back chair with your lower back up against the chair. Lean forward as if to engage. Be aware of your physiology. Feel what you feel. Now think of a number of mildly anxious experiences and fully associate with them. As you relive those experiences, see what you see, hear what you hear, feel what you feel.

Stand up and walk around the room or sing the National Anthem at the top of your voice to break state.

Now sit back against the chair, hips forward, and breathe deeply. Press your shoulders back, relax and allow them to sit in their natural comfortable position. Drop your chin and ensure your head is in line with your shoulders. Allow your eyes to lose focus.

As you now think about those experiences that are moderately uncomfortable, imagine that you are taking yourself out of your body and are seeing yourself in this experience from a distance.

Take yourself even further into the distance and see how you feel now. Now take yourself a hundred feet up in the air and look down on the experience. How is it different now? How do the two positions feel different?

If you find yourself associating with a negative event or memory begin by changing your physiology – adopt a posture that encourages you to dissociate.

EXERCISE FOUR – WATCH WITHOUT FEAR

You can train yourself to automatically distance yourself from a given situation. One way to do this is through the use of imagery. Take yourself back to the uncomfortable experience that you were thinking about in the previous exercise. Now imagine a smokescreen partially obscuring your picture of the experience. If the experience still feels painful, make the smokescreen thicker or darker.

EXERCISE FIVE – PUT IT IN REVERSE

The next time a traumatic memory comes up, stay with it instead of trying to push it away. As the experience comes up, float up out of your self and imagine that you are watching the situation from a hundred foot up in the air. See what there is to learn about the experience from this dissociated perspective. What healing words of wisdom would you say to yourself to help yourself heal from the trauma of this event? Imagine a powerful white healing light and at the end of the situation, imagine that you jump into it with that light and are being sucked backwards through the event by a giant vacuum at great speed – this takes just a second. Now take yourself to before the experience happened. As you think about the experience now how is it different? Do this as many times as it takes to completely neutralize the experience.

EXERCISE SIX – ALTER YOUR VIEW

DO THE TRAUMA ALGORITHM (see page 118) BEFORE DOING THIS EXERCISE.

Now put yourself into self-hypnosis.

As you relax deeper and deeper you recognize that although you cannot change what happened in the past, your subconscious mind has the most incredible ability to change the way that you feel about it now. Having performed the appropiate TFT exercise you begin to feel so different about the experience. From now on your subconscious mind works powerfully for you so that any emotions concerning this event seem less and less and you find yourself so much more relaxed within yourself, so much more comfortable about the past. You are able now to begin the process of simply letting go of any old emotions that are no longer useful to you. Imagine now that you are sitting in the middle of a cinema with a giant movie screen in front.

Imagine floating to the projection booth. As you find yourself in the projection booth you feel so much more detached and you feel comfortable about playing the movie of the experience that, in the past, caused you distress. By your side is a set of controls that allow you to change the experience. Now, as you watch this experience, use those controls so that all the colours seem to fade and the experience seems to happen in black and white. The picture seems to become less important and, as it now begins to shrink, you press the button that changes the sound in a way that suits you better. Now, as you watch and hear this movie, you think of some resources that would have been useful to you in this experience – perhaps strength, perhaps self-love. The screen becomes clear now as your subconscious mind searches to find references of those experiences in your mind. Now play the movies of those experiences up on the screen. Now take all the good qualities from these experiences, bring the other picture back and give it those new qualities. Mix them in now with the changes that you have already made so that you now begin to see yourself responding differently. With these resources, hear yourself reacting in a more calm, comforting way. You recognize that you are now beginning to feel differently about that situation. You can now tell yourself 'I am fine, I have survived and I am going to be fine'. You feel a sense of being more resourced for the future and able to let go of the past. You now make a decision to practise this exercise whenever you feel that you need it.

A Final Word –
Lifestyle, Drugs and a Few of My Favourite Remedies

In addition to tackling your anxiety directly through using language, hypnosis and TFT, there are a number of other tools that can be a valuable addition to your toolbox. One of the most simple and effective is exercise.

EXERCISE

If you could bottle the benefits of exercise you could make a fortune. However, whilst its physical benefits are extremely well documented, the beneficial effects it has on the psyche are less well publicized. Exercise releases hormones that affect your mood, reducing anxiety levels and promoting a more relaxed, positive frame of mind. It is now thought that exercise has a therapeutic effect and many doctors are prescribing it as a means of coping with anxiety and for confidence and esteem building.

Many experts are currently debating the optimum intensity at which to exercise if you suffer from anxiety. One study from a major university looked at three different groups of people – one worked out at high intensity, another at moderate levels and yet another took no exercise – and came to the conclusion that if you work out at a high intensity this lowers anxiety levels more significantly than if you work out at a moderate level. However, other studies show that working out consistently at a moderate level will bring your anxiety levels down.

I personally recommend that you exercise according to your fitness level. If you are unfit, work out in a moderate way. If you have a high level of fitness then you can work out more intensely. However, no matter what your level of fitness, exercise brings about improvements in self-esteem and self-image and hence raises your confidence levels. Exercise also gives you time out by distracting you from your everyday problems. As you become physically stronger you become mentally stronger too. Both mind and body work together in harmony and exercise will help you move from an anxious, depressed state to one of well-being. You will also find that your brain works more efficiently and you're able to organize and concentrate more effectively.

Benefits of Physical Exercise

1. It produces endorphins – the body's natural 'happy' drugs – and can reduce stress hormones.
2. It promotes the relaxation response in the body.
3. It is also an empowering activity, creating a sense of confidence and self-achievement and, with certain types of exercise, increased social interaction.
4. It improves your grey cells by improving concentration, memory and alertness.
5. It reduces tiredness and improves your ability to sleep.

I recommend that you do at least 30 minutes of activity 5 days a week. Ensure you do activities that embrace the three 'SSSs' – stamina, strength and suppleness. And remember to be consistent – make exercise as habitual as brushing your teeth.

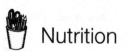 # Nutrition

There is no doubt that faulty diet plays a role in anxiety and depressive illness. The reason for this is straightforward enough – what you eat can have a profound effect on your state of mind. The brain uses a great deal of energy so it is vital that it gets the food it requires. If it doesn't, your attention span, concentration, memory and anxiety levels will all be affected.

The most important brain food is glucose. However, we need to obtain this from appropriate sources. If you eat too many foods that can be quickly converted by the body into glucose – i.e. simple carbohydrates such as sugar and sugary products, honey, some fruits and highly refined cereal products – then you will basically get a 'sugar rush' followed by a slump. And I don't need to tell you what this does for mood and mental wellbeing. Most sugar imbalances in the body are caused by a diet high in these so-called 'simple' carbohydrates. If you suffer from anxiety you need to cut out simple sugars.

Complex Carbohydrates

Instead of getting energy from simple sugars you need to eat plenty of complex carbohydrates such as wholegrains, brown rice, millet, whole-wheat pasta, corn, barley and vegetables. Complex carbohydrates are a better fuel for the body as they are broken down much more slowly and provide a more steady release of energy. Having balanced blood sugar levels is essential for countering states such as depression.

Alcohol and Stimulants

Often when people are anxious they turn to alcohol as a sedative. However, whilst it may help you to achieve a calmer state of mind, it is a means of avoiding problems and can, of course, lead to addiction. Bear in mind too, that alcohol is a source of 'empty' calories because it has very little nutritional value. It also has a diuretic action and a toxic effect on the body. Excess alcohol can cause liver damage, mood swings and an energy imbalance.

When people need a stimulant, rather than a sedative, they often turn to caffeine. If you rely on such things as coffee, tea and certain fizzy drinks to kick your body into action then you may well have exhausted your adrenal glands and are on a vicious cycle of exhaustion and stimulation. Yet another problem with caffeine is that it is addictive, diuretic and is hard on the liver, as it is a toxin. When used excessively, stimulants have a negative effect on your state of mind. Try to stick to no more than one cup of coffee or tea a day. There are a host of caffeine-, sugar- and additive-free drinks on the market. I suggest that you explore these – try herbal teas such as camomile, valerian, peppermint and rose hip. Also drink the recommended eight to ten glasses of water a day.

Food Tips

We are all unique and we all process food differently – one man's meat is indeed another man's poison. I therefore believe that everyone, at some level, would benefit from a personal consultation with a qualified nutritionist, especially those who are are suffering mentally or physically in any way. This is a very valuable investment for your future health and wellbeing. However, there are a number of steps that are broadly recommended for all:

1. If you are suffering from anxiety, you may want to check if you have a sensitivity to certain foods. We tend to be sensitive to the foods that we eat most often, so the most common reactions are to wheat and dairy produce. You can check this either by doing an elimination diet or by being tested.
2. Avoid food that can cause mood swings – coffee, sugar, chocolate and so on.
3. Get your carbohydrate fix from more slowly absorbed complex carbohydrate foods, such as wholegrains and vegetables.
4. Cleanse your body of junk with a good detox programme on a regular basis. Start the day with a cup of boiled water and fresh lemon juice – this is cleansing for the system.
5. Make sure you eat a diet that is balanced, with complex carbohydrates, proteins, fats and loads of vegetables.
6. Occasional sweets are ok. However, if you're prone to mood crashes you need to eat them along with some fibre. This dilutes and absorbs some of the sugar and hence counteracts

the sugar rush and consequent dive in mood it causes.

7. For healthy brain function it is vital to eat monounsaturated fats – so use virgin oil instead of butter. Omega 3 and omega 6 oils – which are found in cold-water fish, oils (flaxseed oil is particularly good) and nuts – are also good for the brain. Avoid saturated fats.

8. B complex vitamins are the main vitamins for the brain and nervous system, so it's advisable to ensure your intake is adequate. Seek advice from your local pharmacist or health shop.

9. Drinking too much alcohol or coffee and tea can deplete vital vitamins and minerals. Too much alcohol in itself causes depression, whilst coffee and tea are stimulants and are best kept to a minimum.

Anti-depressants

Doctors commonly prescribe anti-depressant drugs to counteract anxiety. While there have been many scare stories about them, there is little doubt that they have helped many millions of people. Anti-depressants relieve the symptoms of anxiety and restore the chemical balance in the brain, hence they can help you to cope better – they can give you more energy, help you to sleep and, in general, help you feel better.

Having taken a number of years to come off anti-depressants I was opposed to them for some time. However, having seen so many people suffering from anxiety and depression, I now feel strongly that they play an important role as a *short-term* solution in helping someone who is anxious or depressed cope with life. In the long term it is better for the individual to resolve their issue and seek other ways to find balance. This process, however, should begin while you are on anti-depressants, because the drug itself creates what can be described as a 'buffer' in the mind and this can give you space to think before you react in your old habitual way. You can then begin to experience the effects of behaving differently. Undergoing whatever therapy you feel is appropriate should not be put off until you come off anti-depressants – see them as an aid not a crutch.

Side-effects

Anti-depressants can, of course, have side-effects. These can include dryness of the mouth, constipation, difficulty passing urine, a change in appetite and weight gain. They can also affect sexual functioning. If you suffer from a number of side-effects then do ask your doctor if you can try another type – there are many available and there may well be one that is more suited to you.

Speaking from personal experience, if you are taking anti-depressants I would recommend that you never just come off them. If you do, you're likely to experience withdrawal symptoms. Work with your doctor and give yourself a period of time to reduce the dosage. Seek help and find solutions to whatever comes up as you come off them, whether it is physical, mental or emotional. And make sure you feel a sense of balance before you reduce the quantity further.

Complementary Medicine

On the whole, the medical approach to anxiety in the west is one that relies on drug treatment. This is very much in line with the traditional western approach of seeing the mind and body as separate. In contrast, complementary medicine presupposes that mind, body and spirit are connected; hence it encompasses numerous therapies and medical treatments to address all aspects of our lives. The list below outlines therapies that work well with anxiety disorders:

Hypnotherapy, acupuncture, Neuro Linguistic Programming, acupressure, homeopathy, herbal medicine, Bach flower remedies, Reiki healing, energy healing, meditation, nutrition, Applied Kinesiology, osteopathy, chiropractic treatment, thought field therapy, counselling, cognitive behavioural therapy, reflexology, Ayurvedic medicine, massage.

Nature's Own Pharmacy

There is also a host of natural remedies that can have a powerful effect on our state of mind. Valerian is my favourite. This calm, relaxing (though very smelly) herb is an excellent aid for promoting calm and a good night's sleep. Kava – made from the root of a Polynesian pepper tree – also has calming effects, as does lavender. Chamomile is excellent for relieving tension and anxiety; St Johns Wort is useful for depression; passionflower is said to have relaxing qualities, both physically and mentally; and skullcap is good for nervous tension.

The Bach Flower Remedies

One of my favourite therapies, which you can buy over the counter at any health shop or chemist, is the Bach flower remedies. These work extremely well in conjunction with whatever other therapies or medicine you are taking. They are designed to counteract emotional problems and are very much geared to treating the individual as a whole. There are 38 remedies in total but for the purposes of this book we will stick to the ones for fear, lack of confidence and anxiety.

Mimulus: The aim of this herb is to make it easier to face the anxieties of the day. It is suitable for those who know what they are afraid of.

Rock Rose: This translucent yellow plant is for those who have suffered or who are suffering a great terror or are in state of paralysis.

Aspen: This remedy is for free-floating anxieties that seem to come on for no reason whatsoever. If you have fears that are unidentified you should respond well to this herb.

Cherry Plum: The cherry plum remedy is suitable for the fear of loss of reason and self-control.

Red Chestnut: This remedy is for a fear for the wellbeing and safety of someone else.

Star of Bethlehem: This is excellent for shock.

Impatiens: This is suitable for mental stress.

Sleep

Last, but by no means least, comes sleep – a vital tool for counteracting anxiety. Insomnia and a lack of sleep contribute to anxious states of mind. This can make people irritable and anxious and can blow existing anxiety out of all proportion, creating a vicious circle of mental, emotional and physical fatigue.

Everybody's body clock works in different ways. Different people need different amounts of sleep – some need five hours a night others need eight. One of the problems with modern-day living is that our natural sleep patterns are disturbed. It is estimated that 50 per cent of the population constantly wakes up feeling fatigued and a large percentage suffer from insomnia. Your quality of sleep can be affected by a number of factors – poor nutrition, lack of exercise and of course anxious thoughts and high stress levels.

There are numerous remedies on the market, however, I would not recommend sleeping pills if you want a refreshing night's sleep. Instead, try natural remedies such as valerian – there are a number of these remedies out there so experiment with what works best for you.

The tools in this book should also help improve the quality of your sleep. TFT will take the charge out of your anxieties, while self-hypnosis will contribute hugely by making deep relaxation a more familiar state for you. You can also use the power of suggestion during hypnosis to tell yourself that you will sleep well – and of course you can visualize yourself slumbering contentedly.

Regular exercise and addressing your nutritional status will also help. So too will having some form of regular pattern where you wind down for the evening, for instance listening to relaxing music, reading, having a nice relaxing bath or enjoying a relaxing herbal tea.

Oh, and Let's not Forget …

We live in a world that is increasingly isolating us from each other. Numerous studies show that anything that promotes a sense of isolation can lead to physical or mental and emotional malaise. Therefore building a good support network is an important aspect of managing anxiety. If you find yourself more isolated than you care to be, you need to think about redressing the balance by developing new relationships with supportive people who accept you as you are. If you suffer from social anxiety then do the TFT algorithm and exercises prescribed on page 118. If you're not overly fond of people then a pet may be a good idea. The unconditional love that you get and give to animals can be a powerful form of communication.

Having strong spiritual beliefs is also a powerful way of coping with anxiety and depression. Doctors are now encouraging their patients to combat their anxiety through practises such as meditation or prayer. Both of these activities induce the relaxation response in the body.

Studies have shown those individuals with a strong faith or who meditate regularly are less likely to suffer from high blood pressure or depression and are likely to have stronger immune systems and live longer.

I hope that all the tools in this book will prove useful to you in whatever area of your life they are needed. Please pass them on to friends and family so that we can all enjoy an anxiety-free life if we choose.

Good luck
Gloria Thomas

Appendix:
A Letter from Kosovo

November 9, 2001

Dear Colleagues,

Three days ago, I received a letter from Shkelzen Syla, MD, Medical Chief of Staff of all Kosovo. The text is reproduced below.

You may read the background of this letter in the article by Carl Johnson, PhD ABEPP (Clin Psych) and his co-authors in the October issue of the *Journal of Clinical Psychology*. They are: Mustafe Shala, MD, Xhevdet Sejdijaj, MD, Robert Odell, MD, and Kadengjika Dabishevci, MD. Two of the co-authors are with the American Embassy and, as you can see, all of the co-authors are physicians.

The recent October issue is the special issue of the *Journal of Clinical Psychology* where I served as special editor and which presents preliminary research on TFT.

It is important to understand that many of the traumas treated in Kosovo are particularly tragic and unspeakable in their horror.

The letter is now, or soon will be, on our web.

My heartfelt thanks go to Dr Johnson and his colleagues, including Jo Cooper and Ian Graham (both from the UK) who carried out the great work over there. My sincere thanks also to Dr Syla for courageously expressing his views in writing and allowing me to reproduce them.

Roger

ROGER J. CALLAHAN, PHD
FOUNDER, THOUGHT FIELD THERAPY
www.tftrx.com

The Text

Dr Roger Callahan
California
United States of America

Dear Dr Callahan,

Many well-funded relief organizations have treated the post-traumatic stress here in Kosovo. Some of our people had limited improvement but Kosova had no major change or real hope until volunteer American Professor Carl Johnson came to help us with the method that you discovered, Thought Field Therapy.

We referred our most difficult trauma patients to the Professor. The success from TFT was 100% for every patient and they are still smiling until this day.

The Professor has been training our medical personnel in your amazing methods of psychotherapy and we are also having success now. Dr Callahan, Kosova loves Thought Field Therapy.

As Chief of Staff of the Medical Battalion of K.P.C. I have full authority over all medical decisions in Kosova. I am revising this completely and starting a new national program.

The emphasis of the national program will be Thought Field Therapy.

DR SHKELZEN SYLA
CHIEF OF STAFF

CD Track Listing

Bibliography

Books

Bandler, Richard and Macdonald, Will, *An Insider's Guide to Submodalities* (Meta Publications, Inc., 1998)

Butler, Gillian, *Overcoming Social Anxiety and Shyness* (Constable Robinson, 1999)

Callahan, Dr Roger, with Trubo, Richard, *Tapping the Healer Within* (Contemporary Books, 2001)

Carter, Rita, *Mapping the Mind* (Orion, 1998)

Eden, Donna, *Energy Medicine* (Piatkus, 1998)

Goleman, Daniel, *Emotional Intelligence* (Bloomsbury, 1996)

Krasner, A. M., *The Wizard Within: The Krasner Method of Clinical Hypnotherapy* (American Board of Hypnotherapy Press, 1990)

McKenzie, Dr Kwame, *Understanding Depression* (British Medical Association: Family Doctor series, 1999)

Martin, Paul, *The Sickening Mind: Brain, Behaviour, Immunity and Disease* (Flamingo, 1998)

Pert, Candace, *Molecules of Emotion* (Pocket Books, 1997)

Tallis, Dr Frank, *Understanding Obsessions and Compulsion: A Self-Help Manual* (Sheldon Press, 1992)

Tebetts, Charles, *Self-Hypnosis and Other Mind-Expanding Techniques* (Westwood Publishing Company, Inc., 1987)

Thomas, Gloria, *Think Yourself Trim* (Cassell Illustrated, 2003)

Wells, Adrian, *Cognitive Therapy of Anxiety Disorders: A Practical Manual and Conceptual Guide* (University of Manchester/John Wiley and Sons, 1997)

Sources of Statistics

National Institute of Mental Health USA
e-mail: nimhinfo@nih.gov
website: www.nimh.nih.gov

Mind
e-mail: contact@mind.org.uk
website: www.mind.org.uk

Depression Alliance
website: www.depressionalliance.org

National Phobic Society UK
e-mail: nationalphobic@btconnect.com
website: www.phobics-society.org.uk

Further Reading

Butler, Gillian, *Overcoming Social Anxiety and Shyness* (Constable Robinson, 1999)

Callahan, Dr Roger, *Stop the Nightmares of Trauma* (Professional Press, 2000)

—, with Trubo, Richard, Tapping the Healer Within (Contemporary Books, 2001)

Cohen, Pete, *Habit Busting* (Thorsons, 2000)

Ingham, Christine, *Panic Attacks* (Thorsons, 2000)

McDermott, Ian and O'Connor, Joseph, *NLP and Health* (Thorsons, 1996)

Pert, Candace, *Molecules of Emotion* (Pocket Books, 1997)

Shepherd, David, *Presenting Magically* (Crown House Publications, 2001)

Thomas, Gloria, *Think Yourself* series, various authors (Cassell Illustrated)

Weeks, Dr Clare, *Essential Help for Your Nerves* (Thorsons, 2000)

Resources

UK
TFT UK
tel: 0845 458 3225
website: www.thoughtfieldtherapy.co.uk
Lists practitioners and training in the UK

Jo Cooper
PO Box 178
Leicester
LE3 8ZU
tel: 0845 456 9285
e-mail: info@jo-cooper.com
website: www.jo-cooper.com

Depression Alliance UK
35 Westminster Bridge Rd
London
SE1 7JB
tel: 020 7633 0557
website: depresssionalliance.org

The Stress Management Training Institute
Foxhills
30 Victoria Avenue
Shanklin
Isle of Wight
PO37 6LS
tel: 01983 868166
email: admin@smti.org
website: www.smti.org

Mind
15–19 Broadway
London
E15 4BQ
tel: 0845 7660 163 (helpline)
email: contact@mind.org.uk
website: www.mind.org.uk

National Phobics Society
Zion Community Resource Centre
339 Stretford Road
Hulme
Manchester
MI5 4ZY
tel: 0870 770456
e-mail: nationalphobic@btconnect.com
website: www.phobics-society.org.uk

USA
Dr Roger J. Callahan
Callahan Techniques Ltd
Thought Field Therapy Training Center
78–816 Via Carmel
La Quinta
CA 92253
tel: 1 800 359-cure (2873)
tel: +1 (760) 564 1008 (for international enquiries)
website: www.tftrx.com

National Institute for Mental Health
6001 Executive Blvd
Room 8184, Msc 9663
Bethesda
MD 20892-9663

tel: (301) 443 4513 (general enquiries)
e–mail: nimhinfo@nih.gov
website: www.nimh.nih.gov

Anxiety Disorders Association of America
8730 Georgia Avenue Suite 600
Silver Spring
MD 20910
tel: (240) 485–1001
website: www.adaa.org

Freedom from Fear
308 Seaview Avenue
Statten Island
New York
NY 10305
website: www.freedomfromfear.com

Obsessive Compulsive Foundation
337 Notch Hill Road
North Branford
CT 06471
website: www.ocfoundation.org

Australia
Australian Psychological Society
PO Box 38
Flinders Lane
Melbourne
Victoria 8009
tel: 1800 333 497 or 03 8662 3300
e–mail: contactus@psychsociety.com.au
website: www.aps.psychsociety.com.au

Australian Psychological Association
PO Box 422
Erindale Centre
Australian Capital Territory 2903
tel: 02 9990 0490

Association of Private Practising Psychologists
PO Box 157
Paddington
Queensland 4064
tel: 07 3839 0064
Steve Duncan (President)
tel: 07 5526 5432

Australian College of Clinical Psychologists
GPO Box 3008
Canberra 2601
tel: 02 6285 2499
e-mail: secretary@accp.org.au
website: www.accp.org.au

How to Contact the Author

If you wish to contact Gloria Thomas for any of her anxiety or lifestyle packages you can do so through her website: www.reshape.co.uk . You can also write to her at:

The Third Space Medicine
13 Sherwood Street
London
W1F 7BR
United Kingdom
tel: 020 7439 7332

Index